The Natural PHARMACIST™

P9-DHF-309

Inside—Find the Answers to These Questions and More

☑ What are the benefits of the herb kava for anxiety? (See page 63.)

☑ How much should I take—and for how long? (See page 76.)

☑ What form of kava should I take? (See page 77.)

☑ How long do I have to take it before I start seeing results? (See page 79.)

☑ Does kava have any side effects? (See page 87.)

☑ Is kava addictive? (See page 93.)

☑ What standard medications should not be combined with kava? (See page 93.)

☑ Can the herb valerian help my insomnia? (See page 130.)

☑ Can I use melatonin to relieve insomnia? (See page 136.)

☑ How does kava compare to prescription drugs? (See page 99.)

THE NATURAL PHARMACIST Library

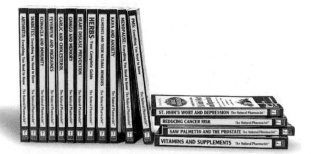

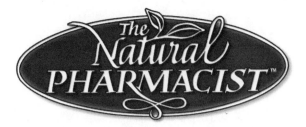

Everything You Need to Know About

Kava and Anxiety

Constance Grauds, R.Ph.

Series Editors

Steven Bratman, M.D.

David Kroll, Ph.D.

A DIVISION OF PRIMA PUBLISHING

Visit us online at www.thenaturalpharmacist.com

Warning—Disclaimer

This book is not intended to provide medical advice and is sold with the understanding that the publisher and the author are not liable for the misconception or misuse of information provided. The author and Prima Publishing shall have neither liability nor responsibility to any person or entity with respect to any loss, damage, or injury caused or alleged to be caused directly or indirectly by the information contained in this book or the use of any products mentioned. Readers should not use any of the products discussed in this book without the advice of a medical professional.

The Food and Drug Administration has not approved the use of any of the natural treatments discussed in this book. This book, and the information contained herein, has not been approved by the Food and Drug Administration.

Pseudonyms are used throughout to protect the privacy of individuals involved.

PRIMA HEALTH and colophon are trademarks of Prima Communications, Inc.

THE NATURAL PHARMACIST™ is a trademark of Prima Communications, Inc.

All products mentioned in this book are trademarks of their respective companies.

Illustrations by Helene D. Stevens and Gale Mueller. Illustrations © 1999 Prima Publishing. All rights reserved.

Library of Congress Cataloging-in-Publication Data

Grauds, Constance.
    Kava and anxiety / Constance Grauds.
       p.   cm.—(The natural pharmacist)
    Includes bibliographical references and index.
    ISBN 0-7615-1613-1
    1. Anxiety—Alternative treatment.   2. Kava (Beverage)—Therapeutic use.
    3. Kava plant—Therapeutic use.   4. Herbs—Therapeutic use.   I. Title.   II. Series.
    RC531.G73   1999
    616.85'22306—dc21   98-43577
                                                                                          CIP

                    00 01 02 HH 10 9 8 7 6 5 4 3 2
                    Printed in the United States of America

Visit us online at www.thenaturalpharmacist.com

Contents

What Makes This Book Different?

The interest in natural medicine has never been greater. According to the National Association of Chain Drug Stores, 65 million Americans are using natural supplements, and the number is growing! Yet, it is hard for the consumer to find trustworthy sources for balanced information about this emerging field. Why? Frankly, natural medicine has had a checkered history. From snake oil potions sold at the turn of the century to those books, magazines, and product catalogs that hype miracle cures today, this is a field where exaggerated claims have been the norm. Proponents of natural medicine have tended to abuse science, treating it more as a marketing tool than a means of discovering the truth.

But there is truth to be found. Studies of vitamins, minerals, and other food supplements have been with us since these nutritional substances were first discovered, and the level and quality of this science has grown dramatically in the last 20 years. Herbal medicine has been neglected in the United States, but in Europe, this, the oldest of all healing arts, has been the subject of tremendous and ongoing scientific interest.

At present, for a number of herbs and supplements, it is possible to give reasonably scientific answers to the questions: How well does this work? How safe is it? What types of conditions is it best used for?

THE NATURAL PHARMACIST series is designed to cut through the hype and tell you what we know and what we don't know about popular natural treatments. These books are more conservative than any others available, more honest about the weaknesses of natural approaches, more fair in their comparisons of natural and conventional treatments. You won't find any miracle cures here, but you will discover useful options that can help you become healthier.

Why Choose Natural Treatments?

Although the science behind natural medicine continues to grow, this is still a much less scientifically validated field than conventional medicine. You might ask, "Why should I resort to an herb that is only partly proven, when I could take a drug with solid science behind it?" There are at least three good reasons to consider natural alternatives.

First, some herbs and supplements offer benefits that are not matched by any conventional drug. Vitamin E is a good example. It appears to help prevent prostate cancer, a benefit that no standard medication can claim. Also, vitamin E almost certainly helps prevent heart disease. While there are standard drugs that also prevent heart disease, vitamin E works differently and may be able to complement many of the other approaches.

Another example is the herb milk thistle. Studies strongly suggest that this herb can protect the liver from injury. There is no pill or tablet your doctor can prescribe to do the same.

Even if the science behind some of these treatments is less than perfect, when the risks are low and the possible benefit high, a natural treatment may be worth trying. It is a little-known fact that for many conventional treatments the science is less than perfect as well, and physicians must balance uncertain benefits against incompletely understood risks.

A second reason to consider natural therapies is that some may offer benefits comparable to those of drugs with fewer side effects. The herb St. John's wort is a good example. Reasonably strong scientific evidence suggests that this herb is an effective treatment for mild to moderate depression, while producing fewer side effects on average than conventional medications. Saw palmetto for benign enlargement of the prostate, ginkgo for relieving symptoms and perhaps slowing the progression of Alzheimer's disease, and glucosamine for osteoarthritis are other examples. This is not to say that herbs and supplements are completely harmless—they're not—but for most the level of risk is quite low.

Finally, there is a philosophical point to consider. For many people, it "feels" better to use a treatment that comes from nature instead of from a laboratory. Just as you might rather wear all-cotton clothing than polyester, or look at a mountain landscape rather than the skyscrapers of a downtown city, natural treatments may simply feel more compatible with your view of life. We can quibble endlessly about just what "natural" means and whether a certain treatment is "actually" natural or not, but such arguments are beside the point. The difference is in the feeling, and feelings matter. In fact, having a good feeling about taking an herb may lead you to use it more consistently than you would a prescription drug.

Of course, at times synthetic drugs may be necessary and even lifesaving. But on many other occasions it may be quite reasonable to turn to an herb or supplement instead of a drug.

To make good decisions you need good information. Unfortunately, while hundreds of books on alternative medicine are published every year, many are highly misleading. The phrase "studies prove" is often used when the studies in question are so small or so badly conducted that they prove nothing at all. You may even find that the "data" from other books comes from studies with petri dishes and not real people!

You can't even assume that books written by well-known authors are scientifically sound. Many of these authors rely on secondary writers, leading to a game of "telephone," where misconceptions are passed around from book to book. And there's a strong tendency to exaggerate the power of natural remedies, whitewashing them with selective reporting.

THE NATURAL PHARMACIST series gives you the balanced information you need to make informed decisions about your health needs. Setting a new, high standard of accuracy and objectivity, these books take a realistic look at the herbs and supplements you read about in the news. You will encounter both favorable and unfavorable studies in these pages and will learn about both the benefits and the risks of natural treatments.

THE NATURAL PHARMACIST series is the source you can trust.

Steven Bratman, M.D.
David Kroll, Ph.D.

Introduction

Some 50 million Americans suffer from anxiety. The poet W. H. Auden wrote in 1948 that modern people were living in "the age of anxiety." At the end of the twentieth century, we are more anxious than ever. Modern life, with its stresses and pressures, leaves us little peace and quiet in which to make sense of the rapidly changing world we live in. We rush from job to errands to home and back again, until the stress begins to take its toll. Anxiety is a normal reaction to stress, but it can grow into a debilitating problem that interferes with our personal and professional lives.

For most of the twentieth century, anxiety has been treated with either psychotherapy or strong sedative drugs, or a combination of the two. Psychotherapy can be very helpful, but unfortunately it can require a lot of time as well as money. Many people suffer from anxiety precisely because they don't have enough time (or money) to begin with!

Medications have been a very popular way to treat anxiety. At their best, medications can relieve the painful, troubling feelings of anxiety while the sufferer learns how to reduce the sources of anxiety in his or her life. The type of drugs used for much of this century were barbiturates—powerfully sedating medications that tended to leave people feeling drowsy and "drugged." Barbiturates could be dangerously addictive, and an overdose could be fatal. While these medications could relieve painful feelings of anxiety, they also made it difficult to carry on a healthy life at work and at home.

In the 1960s, medical treatment for anxiety advanced with the discovery of the benzodiazepine drugs, such as Valium and Librium. They became the sought-after panacea for millions of Americans because they were less sedating than barbiturates, less addictive, and seldom caused death from overdose. They were also very effective in relieving the feelings of anxiety, yet these medications also had potentially troubling side effects, including drowsiness and addiction. Even an effective medication can become a crutch if it takes the place of real, holistic change to address the source of anxiety in one's life. Today there is a much stronger interest in holistic medicine, which aims to treat the whole person rather than just the symptoms. A holistic treatment for anxiety might involve a combination of medication, relaxing exercises, changes in diet or lifestyle, and/or psychotherapy. There is also an interest in natural, gentle alternatives to drugs.

One leading natural treatment for anxiety today is kava, a South Pacific herb that has been used as an antianxiety treatment first in Europe and now in North America as well. The Europeans learned about kava from the indigenous peoples of the South Pacific islands, who traditionally have used it as a beverage to promote relaxation and camaraderie. There is good evidence suggesting that kava is an effective treatment for anxiety. Although it seems to be less powerful than the benzodiazepine drugs, kava seems to leave many people feeling alert rather than drowsy, and there have been no problems with addiction reported.

Kava is currently being studied, and more research is needed. There is much that we don't yet know about how it works and how it can be used most effectively. It's not a panacea—no herbal or pharmaceutical treatment is—but it appears to be a gentle, effective alternative for many people who suffer from generalized anxiety. (It is probably not strong enough to treat severe anxiety disorders.)

This book will give you a fair appraisal of kava's strengths and weaknesses, as well as an objective comparison between kava and conventional drugs. We've examined the evidence, and present it here to help you decide whether this herb might be useful for you.

What Is Kava?

T he kava plant is a hearty perennial shrub with large heart-shaped leaves (see figure 1). It belongs to the pepper family (*Piperaceae*) and thrives in the tropical islands of the South Pacific—Hawaii, New Guinea, Fiji, Tonga, Tahiti, Micronesia, and Samoa—where it can grow up to 9 feet tall. Used as a brew and, more recently, as a natural herbal remedy, kava promotes friendliness and sociability, produces relaxing sensations (physical as well as mental), and reduces anxiety and muscle tensions. Its effects can be described as ranging from mildly sedating to mildly intoxicating, depending on the dose.

It seems almost too much of a coincidence that kava originated in the island paradises where so many travelers have sought peace and tranquility. Indeed, the inhabitants of these islands have used kava for centuries as a relaxing social drink; perhaps this custom is partly responsible for the image we have today of the South Pacific islands as peaceful, friendly places. Kava has been cultivated by the

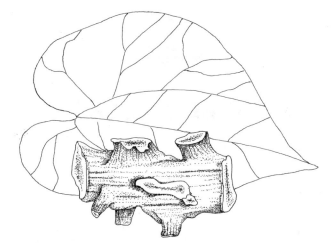

Figure 1. *Kava leaf and root*

inhabitants of these islands so long that it has become dependent on human care and cannot grow on its own.

Many types of kava plants are cultivated, but the most desired are the so-called black (purple) and white (light-green) types. With a short (2½- to 3-year) growing season and a high resistance to disease, the black type is preferred by growers. The white type is considered more potent and thus is preferred by users.

The medicinally active part of the kava plant is the root, which grows to a large size—the roots of a plant less than 1 year old can weigh more than 2 pounds. Heavily knotted roots are especially prized for their supposed extra flavor and strength.

Like most herbal roots, kava has a strong but pleasant "earthy" odor and flavor. Kava produces a tingling, numbing sensation in the mouth on direct contact. Island kava drinkers make kava into a relaxing beverage by steeping the mashed root in cold water. In Europe and the United

States, people who enjoy its taste can obtain kava in tea, beverage, and tincture forms. For those who don't like the taste of kava, tablets and capsules are now available as well. (For more about the different forms of kava see chapter 6.)

Why Is It Called Kava?

Captain Cook was one of the first Europeans to describe kava use. In 1770, Cook's botanist, J. G. A. Forster, gave kava its scientific name, *Piper methysticum,* meaning "intoxicating pepper." The kava plant is closely related to the pepper plant, and the Greek word *methustikos* means "intoxicating drink."

The common name *kava,* or *kava-kava,* and its variants *kawa, 'ava,* and *'awa* have long been used in the South Pacific to represent both the plant and the beverage made from it. There are many kinds of kava plants and many different names for kava. For example, *liwa* is the name for a variation of kava with short joints and green stalks, and *papa* is the

The medicinally active part of the kava plant is the root, which grows to a large size—the roots of a plant less than 1 year old can weigh more than 2 pounds.

name for a kava with short joints and spotted stalks. *Marea* kava has a root with a lemon-yellow interior.

What Is in Kava?

The known active components of kava are a group of fat-soluble compounds, called *kavalactones*, that make up

Nomenclature

In traditional South Pacific island use, certain types of kavas are reserved for special occasions. For example, certain *liwa* and *papa* kinds are used only for the gods and ceremonial affairs. A tall kava plant with pale-green joints and dark-green spots, called *taramaete,* is specifically reserved for sacrifices to the gods.

Another naming system is based on differences in the effects of kava plants on the mind and body. For example, *melmel,* meaning "nothing," is so named because of its weak effects. *Tudei,* meaning "two day," produces highly potent kava with long-lasting effects. The reportedly aphrodisiac effects of another type of kava with red stems and light-colored leaves are reflected in its name *avini,* which means "pleasure."

from 3 to 20% of the rootstock, depending on the age and type of the plant. These kavalactones, exert subtle effects on the nervous system. Kava roots range in color from white to dark yellow, depending on the concentration of kavalactones; the darker the root, the greater the concentration of kavalactones.

There are different types of kavalactones. The major kavalactones include dihydrokavain, kavain, methysticin, and dihydromethysticin. Kavalactones have been isolated and studied, and it is well established that these compounds have mild sedative effects. Less research has been done on the effects of the whole kava plant. We don't know whether there are other active chemicals in the kava plant or whether a combination of all the chemicals found in the whole plant might contribute to the effects that people experience when taking kava.

Nothing but the Best

Natives of the South Pacific use systematic gardening pro-cedures to ensure that only preferred types of kava are grown. If the user does not like the effects of the drink pre-pared from a certain root, the stems are allowed to wither and die. Thus, indigenous cultures have maintained an intimate knowledge of the subtle variations of kava and its effects on the body and mind.

Islanders' naming of kava types (based on *visible* dif-ferences in the plant), has recently been proven to reflect underlying *chemical* differences—kavalactone concentra-tions actually differ among the variously named plant types.

The age of the root makes a big difference in potency. The concentration of kavalactones in the root increases as the root increases in size and weight. The most desirable kava roots are not mature enough for drinking until 5 or more years of age, and for special events native kava growers put aside a few of their prized 10- or 15-year-old plants.

Kavalactones have been isolated and studied, and it is well established that these com-pounds have mild sedative effects.

What Was Kava Used for Historically?

Captain Cook and the early eighteenth-century Dutch traders were the first Europeans to see and record the uses of kava. In 1773, on their second Pacific voyage off the west coast of Tahiti, Cook and his crew were offered kava by local natives who used it as an integral part of religious and everyday life. The ritual wasn't all that different from sharing a pot of tea. However, when Christian missionaries arrived on the islands, they saw it a bit differently. To them, the daily kava-drinking ceremony at sunset, signaling the end of the workday, was a heathen practice that ran contrary to biblical teachings. The missionaries waged a number of campaigns to eradicate kava drinking that ranged from prohibition to harassment of those who practiced the local religion.

Today, the Christian church's opposition to kava among these islands has long since ended, and both natives and government officials drink kava in honor of traditional customs and to relax at the end of the day.

In addition to kava's uses for religious and social ceremonial purposes, the plant has a long-standing and widespread history as an herbal medicine throughout the South Pacific islands. These islanders have used kava as a sedative and an aphrodisiac and to treat venereal diseases, wounds, headaches, colds, inflammations of the uterus, and rheumatism. Hawaii's kahunas also used kava to restore strength to weary muscles and to treat stomach ailments, colds, urinary difficulties, headaches, asthma, and rheumatism.

Historically, kava has been of little economic importance (in terms of importing and exporting), because it was used mainly as a local beverage. However, in recent decades it has become popular in Europe as a *phytomedicine* (plant-based medicine) for anxiety. The demand in the United States is also increasing. Because of increased demand, kava is becoming an important cash crop for Pacific islanders as an international export.

Kava's Entry into Modern Medicine

The first serious research of the possible medicinal use of kava began in the 1850s and 1860s in Europe (mainly in

Ceremonial Usage

Present-day ceremonies of welcome in Tonga, Samoa, and Fiji always include kava. President and Mrs. Lyndon Johnson were offered the kava drink on their visit to Samoa. Queen Elizabeth of Great Britain and members of the royal family, Pope John Paul II, and First Lady Hillary Rodham Clinton have partaken of kava during their visits to Fiji, where kava continues to occupy a central, although somewhat diminished, place in both the special events and the everyday lives of the islanders.

Germany). Scientists learned to make extracts into pills, tinctures, and syrups which were used medicinally as sedatives, tranquilizers, muscle relaxants, as well as a treatment for menopausal symptoms and urinary tract and bladder disorders. By 1914, kava had made its way into the *British Pharmacopoeia;* by 1920, kava appeared in European dispensaries as a sedative and high-blood-pressure medicine. By 1950, the *U.S. Pharmacopoeia* listed kava as a treatment for nervous disorders and urogenital tract irritations. However, shortly thereafter, in the United States, kava (as well as most other medicinal herbs) fell into disfavor as synthetic pharmaceuticals gained popularity. Some European countries, to the contrary, continued to use kava and other botanical medicines in their health-care system.

Today, more than a dozen medicinal products derived from kava are available on the European market. In Germany, the official governmental body that regulates herbs (known as Commission E) approves the use of kava for the treatment of "states of nervous anxiety, tension, and agitation." Some evidence suggests that it may be specifically helpful for the anxiety associated with menopause (see chapter 5 for more information). In France, kava is also recognized by health officials for the treatment of urinary tract infections.

Even though kava is well recognized and widely used by doctors in Europe for the treatment anxiety, insomnia, and other health problems, in the United States, kava currently remains the province of alternative medicine. As a pharmacist, I encourage you to read this entire book (especially chapter 7, which deals with kava's potential toxicity and side effects), before deciding to take kava.

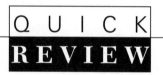

QUICK REVIEW

- Historically, kava (*Piper methysticum*) has been used as a relaxing drink in the cultures of the South Pacific islands.

- In Hawaii and other South Pacific islands today, sharing a bowl or a cup of kava is still a stress-relieving ritual that fosters socializing and friendship.

- Kava is specifically approved in Germany for the treatment of anxiety and nervous tension. It's also used for the same purpose in many other European countries, and increasingly so in the United States as well.

- Some evidence suggests that kava may be specifically helpful for anxiety related to menopause.

- Kava's effects range from mildly sedative to mildly intoxicating depending on the dose.

- Before deciding to use kava, please make sure to read about possible safety issues in chapter 7.

The Symptoms
of Anxiety

This chapter describes the symptoms of anxiety, from the mildest to the most severe. Different treatments might be more or less useful, depending on the type of anxiety. Before we go on to consider the strengths and weaknesses of the available treatments for anxiety, we need to consider the many types and degrees of anxiety.

The word *anxiety* means different things to different people. I like to think of anxiety as two different words: anxiety with a small "a" and Anxiety with a big "A." The average person usually accepts anxiety as part of the give-and-take of everyday life. "Hey, we all have problems, right? So, get over it!" This is anxiety with a small "a." It usually has an obvious and even mundane cause, for example, a flooded basement or a sick child. We all have our own ways of addressing these causes. Sometimes we confront an issue head-on, sometimes we run away, and sometimes we just sit and cry. Human solutions to problems seem to run the gamut of all possible extremes. Most would agree that our unique solutions to such problems make life more interesting in the long run.

When we are anxious, the body's famous "fight-or-flight" response comes into play. This response consists of our sympathetic nervous system pumping out a chemical called *adrenaline,* which raises blood pressure and speeds up the heart rate; breathing becomes more rapid, and we sweat, all to prepare the body for a burst of energy and possibly for becoming wounded. This biological reaction prepares us for possible danger by giving us the energy we need to either fight or run.

> **Generalized anxiety disorder (GAD) is anxiety that has taken on a life of its own.**

The fight-or-flight response is ideally suited to extreme physical dangers. It no doubt made our ancestors better able to run away from cave bears. However, most situations in modern daily life are not really life threatening, although sometimes we might think they are. Every day we face many stressful situations that don't require an all-or-nothing physical response, but our bodies still react as they've been doing for millions of years. To our bodies, sometimes the car that just cut us off on the freeway seems more like a lion threatening the lives of our children.

Fortunately, most us can moderate our fight-or-flight instincts into appropriate responses, such as heightened awareness and focus. For example, our anxiety over an upcoming test causes us to study harder, or the tension caused by heavy traffic increases our awareness for quicker reaction times. Our concern for loved ones insists that we call them regularly. Such feelings and thoughts come and go as a part of our daily routine. Our instinctive coping skills alert us to what must be done to handle the situation effectively, and we accept this mild anxiety as normal.

However, for some of us, worry and fear dominate life. Everyday existence is a baffling and frustrating struggle against overwhelming feelings that seem to be out of proportion to the actual danger at hand. These feelings can't be willed away, even if the individual suffering from them knows that they're excessive. This is the normal fight-or-flight response taken to an extreme—Anxiety with a big "A." Technically, it's called generalized anxiety disorder (GAD), which is anxiety that has taken on a life of its own, become constant, "free-floating anxiety," as it's sometimes called. Perhaps 2 to 3% of people in the United States alone suffer from this disease. "I feel like the axe is about to fall any minute," said one woman with a moderately severe case of GAD, "like I'm about to lose my job, or get arrested, or something is about to happen to my daughter. None of that is really happening, and I know it, but I'm scared about it just the same."

Constant muscle tension, apprehensive expectation, constant vigilance against a nonspecific threat, restlessness, irritability, difficulty concentrating, and a tendency to break into a sweat or a heart-pounding throb of fear are some of the symptoms of GAD. Occasionally, panic attacks can develop, although not as frequently as in true panic disorder (discussed in more detail later in this chapter). We don't know what causes GAD, but it seems to be more than simply an accumulation of stresses. Something has shifted in the mind—the "warning" switch is always on.

Constant anxiety is debilitating and can lead to depression, or, in an attempt to escape from it, people can turn to alcohol or drugs. Although psychotherapy is a much better answer, when anxiety is severe, it may not be enough. "I'm too nervous to pay attention to what my therapist is saying,"

Sharon's Story

Sharon is a 35-year-old mother of two children. When her mother had a severe stroke at age 65, Sharon was surprised by the intensity of her reaction. "Mom was always the strong one in the family. I guess I took her for granted, and when she was suddenly frail and needed my help, it really got to me." For a while, it wasn't clear whether her mother would live. Sharon found herself unable to sleep or concentrate on her work. "I was always yelling at my kids, too," she says. "Poor things. They were just as worried about Grandma as I was, but I was yelling at them."

Sharon's doctor prescribed the antianxiety medication Klonopin for her. It made her feel more relaxed, but she experienced some troublesome side effects: She felt unsteady on her legs, and her mind wasn't clear enough for her to do her job. Then she read about kava in a magazine. "The idea ap-

said one young man. Medications, such as those described in chapter 4, are frequently necessary, at least on a short-term basis. Evidence suggests that kava too can be useful (see chapter 5). However, medical supervision is essential when anxiety is severe.

Anxiety: Inside and Out

Most anxiety conditions can be divided into two groups, depending on whether they have an outside cause or an inside cause. Outside influences include situations that threaten our bodies and our life pursuits and that have

pealed to me, but I thought I should ask my doctor first." Her physician was supportive of the idea. He told her how long to wait until the Klonopin was out of her system before starting the herb. "I had a couple of really bad days, but then the kava started to work. Within a week I was sailing smoothly again. I kept on taking the kava until my mom got out of the hospital. Seeing her on her feet again, and her same old self, I didn't need the kava any more."

Sharon would probably be advised to undergo some counseling to prepare her in the event her mother fell ill in the future, but kava got her through a difficult period successfully.

Of course, an anecdote like this doesn't prove that kava is an effective treatment for anxiety. See chapter 5 for a review of the scientific evidence that kava really works.

clearly arisen outside our control. A work-related injury that could jeopardize your health and your job, sickness of a loved one, a financial crisis, or an impending divorce are typical outside causes of anxiety. These are *situational anxieties,* in that they are usually short term and subside once the outside cause is removed. However, sometimes the feelings can be severe enough to interfere with your ability to sleep or cope with the demands of life in the short term.

Another example of anxiety caused by an outside influence is fear about walking past the neighbor's dog that bit you in the past. This kind of anxiety is a natural reaction based on past experience. However, such apprehension can also expand into a fear of all dogs or even of going outside at all. For some people, severe reactions of panic and phobia can be triggered by common external causes.

In contrast to such outside causes, some anxieties seem to have little relationship to external events. A common example of an inside cause of anxiety is fear of abandonment. A person suffering from such anxiety might have no reason to think that his wife wants to leave him, but he still worries constantly. Another common anxiety of this type is a general fear of being disliked. These anxieties with inside causes are especially frustrating because the cause is more difficult to detect than outside causes, such as sudden illnesses in the family, which are more clear. People suffering from an inside cause of anxiety might not know why they're anxious, yet the feelings persist. For some, these inside-caused anxieties can even produce sudden, severe anxiety symptoms or overwhelming panic. Such debilitating attacks usually require professional help.

Stress-Related Anxiety

We live in a fast-paced, complex society that is getting faster and more complex all the time. The computer revolution has increased the pace of our daily lives. News has become instantly available from around the world at any time, whether we want it or not. Communications devices ring, beep, or buzz at us wherever we go. Computer networks provide endless access to everything, anytime, at the touch of a button, and employment ads routinely use buzzwords such as "fast-paced," "energetic," and "multitask environment" to describe the workplace. Modern clichés such as "I want it yesterday!" and "Whatever it takes!" are not always used only half-jokingly. The result of all this is a culture of seemingly endless pressure to do, be, go, earn, answer, call, go away, please come back, and on and on and on. Is it any wonder that we get anxious, that we sometimes worry, feel tension, and even have difficulty functioning?

We aren't wrong to feel anxious and worried at times, but why suffer more than we need to? Anxiety has a purpose, and once that purpose has been served, we don't need it anymore. So, why doesn't it simply go away? Because human be-

Anxiety is meant to be a part of life, not to dominate it.

ings don't work that way. We learn. We form habits. Some of the things we learn are good for us, and some are not. Worry and anxiety are often useful in the short term, but they shouldn't become a way of life. In other words, anxiety is meant to be a part of life, not to dominate it.

Generalized Anxiety Disorder

All psychological disorders resemble normal states taken to an extreme. Generalized anxiety disorder (GAD), as we briefly discussed, is a perfect example. Although we all experience stress, with GAD, anxiety is a constant source of pain. GAD sufferers have the feelings of normal anxiety but without an apparent cause.

Fortunately, GAD is generally treatable. However, you should start by seeking professional guidance. Sometimes, anxiety symptoms can be due to another emotional disorder, such as depression, or even a physical illness. Anyone experiencing severe or persistent anxiety should get a full medical evaluation. Kava can be useful as part of an overall treatment plan, but don't combine kava on your own with prescription medications. Such combinations can be dangerous. (For more information on kava and safety, see chapter 7.)

Psychological Symptoms of Anxiety

The symptoms described in the following sections can occur in any form of anxiety, from the mildest to the most severe. If you recognize yourself in these descriptions, kava might be a useful option for you. However, you should consult a physician or other health professional about any anxiety symptoms that are severe; you might be suffering from GAD or another serious condition. Professional guidance is necessary in such cases.

Excessive Worry

According to the *American Heritage Dictionary*, one meaning of *worry* is "To seize with the teeth and shake or tug at repeatedly." When we are worried, we say that something is "gnawing" at us, and it often feels as if a problem has gripped us in its teeth. Worry, then, is a kind of anxiety that is focused on a particular thing, person, or situation that has somehow gotten a grip on us. Although we try, we can't shake it off. Worry makes us unsure and uneasy or even obsessed. All the "what ifs"—"What if it doesn't happen?" "What if he doesn't?" "What if he won't . . ." are simply mind chatter that clogs our thoughts and makes it hard to think clearly and calmly. In fact, excessive worry is part of the clinical definition of anxiety.

Most of us are prone to worry about stressful situations from time to time. A new job with increased responsibilities can trigger an anxious week of anticipation: "What if I can't do it?" we ask ourselves. "I'll really look like a fool!" For most of us, this reaction is normal, however unpleasant it might be. Usually, we begin the new job, learn our duties, adjust to new conditions, and forget that uncomfortable week of anxiety.

However, the worry doesn't always go away. Sometimes it continues to build until it feels out of control. It can grow, like a snowball rolling downhill, as imagined problems build on one another until the worry begins to fill our lives. Excessive or chronic worry can seriously hamper our ability to make decisions and carry them out or even to handle our practical responsibilities.

As we'll see in chapter 5, kava can be helpful in reducing excessive worry. However, if worry becomes a constant, disabling presence, you should seek professional guidance.

Uneasiness and Jitters

Uneasiness is the vague feeling that something isn't right. For some people, it's far more than an occasional reaction to strange or upsetting circumstances; it's a constant, pervasive feeling. This kind of uneasiness makes living every day slightly uncomfortable, unsure and ill at ease, but with no real apparent reason. People suffering from this kind of anxiety might become suspicious of various things, places, or people in their lives in an attempt to locate the source of the uneasiness, but it's elusive. The other shoe never drops, and the feeling of nervous anticipation doesn't go away.

It's natural to be uneasy sometimes, for example, when you walk through a poorly lit parking garage late at night. However, if you feel this way much of the time and out of proportion to the situation at hand, you might be suffering from an anxiety disorder. Psychotherapy, possibly accompanied by medications or kava, can help you relieve persistent uneasiness.

Fear

Fear is so much a part of the human experience that it seems almost unnecessary to describe it here. The important thing to realize is that some fear is normal and appropriate some of the time but never all of the time.

The media today celebrate the fictional exploits of tough, hardened, unstoppable heroes who stare death (and worse) in the eye with scarcely any sign of fear. Their stories can be great fun to watch if you like them; however, the heroes and the situations they face are one-dimensional.

Unlike fictional characters, all real human beings experience fear and its effects at some point in their lives. The fear can be slight, as when someone surprises us by jumping out from behind a door and yelling "Boo!" or it can be intense, such as that experienced by soldiers in war or victims of violent crime. For some people, fear becomes something more than this natural reaction to the world around us. Chronic, extreme fear can be painful and debilitating and can lead to panic and phobic disorders, as we'll discuss at the end of this chapter. We can become fearful of lots of things. We can even become fearful of fear or of life itself. At that point we need to recognize the significance of this potent emotion and find appropriate help.

Heart Palpitations, Pounding, and Racing

Normally, most of us pay little attention to our heartbeat, except during especially heavy exercise or other strenuous physical activity. The heart beats away as regular as a clock—or so we think. Actually, a normal heartbeat is not always regular; it can vary slightly over time, but we're usually not aware of these variations.

The biochemical reactions of anxiety can influence the heart. Anxiety can raise our adrenaline levels, causing our hearts to race, as in the fight-or-flight reaction, or suddenly the heart can seem to pound or "skip" a beat or give us a "double beat," as in palpitations. Heart palpitations or a racing heart can be an unnerving experience, especially for someone who feels anxious to begin with. Changes of heart rate or heartbeat might simply be symptoms of anxiety that will return to normal as anxiety levels are reduced. However, they might also be symptoms of underlying heart problems. If you suffer from heart palpitations or other changes in rhythm or rate, you should check with your physician to ensure that you don't have heart disease.

Stage Fright

Many people become very nervous before appearing in public to make a speech or give a performance. Even famous actors have been known to fall prey to stage fright. Those who experience debilitating stage fright often ask their physicians for a prescription for Inderal (propranolol), a medication that brings down the blood pressure and slows the heart rate. Although effective for some, Inderal and similar blood-pressure-reducing medications can decrease the blood pressure too much, thereby causing weakness and dizziness. The herb valerian (described in chapter 9) might be helpful.

Chest Tightness and Rapid Breathing

Take a moment right now to notice how you are breathing. When relaxed, we breathe slowly and deeply. When anxious, stressed out, or afraid, we tend to breathe ineffectively in short, shallow breaths that move our upper chest but not our abdomen. This is because the extra adrenaline pumped out causes our chest and stomach to tense up. We can't seem to catch our breath. Overbreathing in this way produces more oxygen than the body needs, upsetting the balance of oxygen and carbon dioxide circulating in the blood and throwing several of the body's systems out of balance. This condition, called hyperventilation, is enough in itself to cause anxiety. Anxiety can lead to a vicious cycle in which hyperventilation creates more anxiety and vice versa. Although more common in panic disorder, hyperventilation can also occur in just about anyone during an unusually stressful and anxious day.

A simple remedy for occasional attacks of anxiety-provoked hyperventilation is to breathe into a paper bag to help slow down the intake of oxygen while the body restores balance to its oxygen and carbon dioxide levels. However, be aware that hyperventilation can develop into a habitual pattern, triggered by anxiety and tension, depression, physical and emotional pain, or even tight clothing. Taking note of your breathing throughout the day and during times of stress can help you recognize and improve your breathing patterns. If you're breathing high into your chest with your shoulders heaving constantly throughout the day, try learning to take deep breaths that cause your belly to move. (For further discussion of stress management techniques, see chapter 9.) Keeping anxiety at bay with kava and stress-reducing techniques can help prevent the rapid lung and heart movements that can accompany severe anxiety.

"Butterflies" in the Stomach and Diarrhea

Anyone who has ever given a speech or proposed a marriage knows what "butterflies" in the stomach feel like. For some, these nervous twinges and flutters are rare; for others, they're a normal, everyday occurrence. However, certain stressful situations can turn the butterflies into a queasy stomach, frequent urination, and even nausea or diarrhea. Once again, extra adrenaline pumping during a fight-or-flight reaction causes the body to lighten its load by churning and emptying the bowels, bladder, and stomach.

We've all experienced brief situational stomach jitters from stressful events, and we usually take them in stride as part of the human experience. However, if too many of our days are filled with anxious feelings in the gut that don't resolve themselves with time or antacids, it might be helpful to try some kava. As your high anxiety levels begin to subside with kava, your stomach and intestinal anxiety symptoms may naturally lessen as well. Valerian and lemon balm are other herbs that can be helpful. (For a discussion of valerian and lemon balm, see chapter 9.)

Sweaty and Clammy

Who hasn't heard the expression "I broke out in a cold sweat"? A similar expression is "no sweat," meaning "no problem." To "sweat it" is to worry about something. We have all felt some degree of sweatiness and clamminess when giving a talk, during a job interview, or while on a first date. Anxiety can cause the body to flush and open the sweat glands. This is a normal response that's caused by a flooding of the body with adrenaline and activating the fight-or-flight mode. Sweating naturally cools us down, perhaps as part of the body's preparation for a burst of intense activity. Such a reaction shouldn't surprise or scare us unless it becomes constant or excessive.

This common problem can be dealt with in many ways. The relaxation methods described in chapter 9 can help. Kava might be useful as well.

Tremors, Muscle Tension, and Muscle Aches

Muscle tension is a very common complaint, and it can be one of the first indications of anxiety. The back and neck are especially vulnerable to tension created by posture, behavior, or anxiety. Through muscle tension, our feelings are often reflected in our bodies: When we ache in the mind, we often ache in the body as well. Too often, our bodies reflect the antagonism of our stressful environment as we harden ourselves against a coming "attack." Over time, this reaction becomes habit; it becomes more and more difficult to really relax, and muscle tension becomes muscle pain. Our hands and bodies can actually shake from stress and tension. Body aches and shakiness can be indicators of anxiety. In these cases, relieving the anxiety will often relieve the body pain and tremors. Often, too, the reverse is true; a good body massage does a lot to relieve anxiety.

Kava appears to have some muscle-relaxant and analgesic (painkiller) properties in addition to its antianxiety effects. Pain relief, relaxed muscles, and peace of mind are a godsend for people with symptoms of anxiety. Simply relieving the anxiety with kava might relieve the accompanying body pains naturally, for relaxing the mind automatically relaxes the body.

Muscle tension is a very common complaint, and it can be one of the first indications of anxiety.

We need to be more aware of the stresses in our lives and the psychological postures we adopt to deal with them. Tension can gradually accumulate in our bodies, and, before we realize what's happening, the accumulation can lead us into a classic state of anxiety. Kava can be part of a natural, gentle stress management regimen that can help your poor back and you as well.

Another common result of muscle tension is the so-called charley horse, in which a leg muscle will suddenly seize up in painful constriction, often trembling or shaking uncontrollably. This can sometimes occur during sleep. Leg cramps can be caused by excessive exercise, poor diet, or too much tension. To avoid muscle cramping, make sure to stretch thoroughly before and after exercise and take adequate calcium and magnesium in your daily diet.

Headaches

Headaches are always annoying, but anxiety-related headaches can be debilitating. More than four out of five individuals suffering from chronic anxiety also experience chronic recurrent headaches. The headaches can occur regularly, even daily, and can last for long periods. They can be aggravated by muscle tension, especially in the neck, in turn causing more tension—a vicious cycle of tension and pain.

Cause-and-effect relationships between headaches and stress can be complex. Often, the onset of a new headache indicates the return of anxiety or emotional stress. Indeed, over the long term, treating the headache alone is rarely effective.

Practically everyone has experienced a tension-related headache. The pain is mild to moderate, and the headache is described as having a "tight" quality. These headaches have been known to last anywhere from a few minutes to days or even weeks on end. Symptoms associated with tension-type headaches include dizziness, ringing in the ears, and a blurring of the vision.

More than four out of five individuals suffering from chronic anxiety also experience chronic recurrent headaches.

For some people, such headaches are an everyday occurrence. Often, sufferers are found to have emotional anxieties and psychological causes for their tension. The main features indicating tension-type headaches are tightness or pressure in the muscles around the sides of the head (felt more strongly in the back part of the neck), pain that increases in severity over the course of the day, and headaches that occur after a tense or anxiety-laden situation. It's interesting to note that chronic use of painkillers can actually cause this type of headache and that stopping the drugs can actually relieve them. Also, many people suffering from tension-type headaches respond to antidepressants and antianxiety medications.

Kava, with its muscle-relaxing and anxiety-reducing properties, might be very helpful as well.

Racing Thoughts and Confusion

The mind is a marvelous tool, functioning day and night to give us the information we need to function in the world. Powerful feelings, whether positive or negative, can cloud the mind, a fact to which anyone can attest. Anxiety, too, affects our minds. The racing mind accompanies the racing body in its fight-or-flight reaction as the chemistry of both the body and the mind changes. During extreme anxiety, our minds seem to jump from one thought to another in a quick, chaotic cycle that feels out of control. People say, "I can't seem to collect my thoughts" or "My mind is going a million miles an hour."

During extreme anxiety, our minds seem to jump from one thought to another in a quick, chaotic cycle that feels out of control.

If the anxiety is situational, we usually just sleep it off and start fresh the next day. If we're feeling clouded and confused, the common temptation is to drink coffee in an effort to "clear the head." Caffeine, of course, just makes the anxiety worse. Kava might be a better choice, as might deep breathing or taking a walk.

When racing thoughts and mental confusion last far beyond any normal reaction and interfere with your life, you should seek professional attention. You might be suffering from a severe anxiety disorder or from depression, and psychotherapy as well as medications might be necessary. Kava might also be an option.

Weakness and Fatigue

Anxiety is often accompanied by weakness and fatigue, as our bodies become exhausted from a continual fight-or-flight mode. Weakness and fatigue linked with anxiety is a common experience in the workplace: not the occasional tiredness that comes from working on a tough deadline but chronic, habitual feelings of lethargy and exhaustion. Such fatigue can affect one's attitude toward work and life in general. The same is also often true about the sense of exhaustion from, for example, the anxiety of child care or elder care. I often hear from customers in the pharmacy who complain of being burned out and are looking for a remedy to give them some energy. In all cases, when people come to me with this complaint, I am also immediately concerned that their fatigue might be an indicator of another medical condition, such as diabetes, or a side effect from a medication. It's always good to get to the root of your fatigue before attempting to self-treat. If you usually feel fatigued in the morning, even after getting enough sleep, and the cup of coffee you drink to

Taking kava instead of java might be a better way to find relief from fatigue.

"give you a boost" makes you feel worse, you might be suffering from anxiety. Taking kava instead of java might be a better way to find relief.

Dizziness and Feeling Faint

Most of us have experienced the feeling of being light-headed from standing up too fast, going too long without a meal, or working under the hot sun. We might also experience an occasional feeling of weakness and loss of control when we are feeling overly anxious. These are all normal experiences, but these feelings can also be provoked by excessive anxiety. The adrenaline produced by anxiety causes hyperventilation, then the decreased oxygen and increased carbon dioxide produce dizziness. Contrary to stereotypes, men also faint and experience dizzy spells with anxiety.

If you experience severe, recurring, or unusual spells of dizziness, you should consult your physician to rule out any physical causes.

Dry Mouth and a Lump in the Throat

This is a feeling everyone can relate to: One minute you're fine. The next minute your mouth is so dry that you couldn't lick a stamp to save your life while the officer who's writing you a ticket (or the girl you've just asked to the prom) wonders why you're so quiet. If you've ever tried drinking water in these situations, you've found that it's hard to swallow past the lump in your throat. The extra adrenaline produced during anxious moments dries up saliva and tightens throat muscles. Usually, these feelings go away as soon as the anxiety-provoking moment is past. Dry mouth combined with the muscle tension of anxiety can produce the feeling of a lump in the throat. Practice and training in handling mildly stressful situations, such as public speaking, can help relieve these symptoms. Kava can also help relieve the underlying anxious state.

Feelings of Inadequacy, Embarrassment, and Criticism

So often our failures get the better of us. We try and try, and still the project isn't approved, the attractive person won't return our calls, or everything goes wrong at once. Life is a cycle of ups and downs and is full of little failures. These failures are more embarrassing to us than anyone else. If there is criticism (real or imaginary), we feel inadequate and magnify the perceived criticism even more. Strong emotions can produce anxiety, which tends to isolate and weaken us further. Failure is a fact of life, but sometimes we manufacture imaginary failures within our own anxious minds. Anxious oversensitivity gives rise to feelings of being painfully shy, as if the "whole room is watching me." Such imagined criticism and feelings of inadequacy and embarrassment hamper our life choices and activities.

Low self-esteem interferes with personal relationships and with jobs. We can be our own worse judge and jury. Psychotherapy can help us understand the origin of the inner critic. Sometimes, self-criticism can be so severe and debilitating that medication—mainly antidepressants—is needed to relieve the underlying depression. The herb St. John's wort can also be helpful in cases of mild to moderate depression. (For more on St. John's wort, see *The Natural Pharmacist Guide to St. John's Wort and Depression.*)

Feeling Out of Control

Have you ever been in a situation that started normally in every respect and then, suddenly, seemed to escalate beyond your control, leaving you not knowing what to do? In common parlance, we call this "freaking out" or "losing it." At its worst, this feeling of being out of control can become a panic attack, but we have all experienced lesser degrees of it. The feeling of being out of control comes from the flood of emotions and physical symptoms that accompany anxiety, including fast breathing, rapid heart rate, confusing and racing thoughts, dizziness, and jitters.

Sometimes, people are prone to these feelings because they expect too much order out of life. The reality is that we are never in complete control of anything. We might plan and do the correct things, and we might take the right steps as we know them to be, but life has a way of changing the dance when we least expect it. New coping skills can help us laugh instead of tense up when the dog destroys the sofa or when the child stubbornly insists on having a messy room. Kava can serve as a kind of gentle backup, helping you to relax while you learn better ways to manage your stress. Professional help might be necessary for more extreme forms of these feelings, especially if they develop into full-blown panic attacks.

Feeling Trapped, Isolated, and Rejected

Anxiety is a lonely condition. It tends to make us avoid others or even feel isolated—like a wallflower—in a crowd. Even experiencing mild anxiety, however common, is not a pleasant way to live. Anxiety tends to isolate us from shared human activities. Eventually, our friends and family do what we seem to want; they leave us alone, but then we feel rejected. Soon, we feel trapped by our own high walls—walls that were built for protection but that only make things worse.

If you are feeling alone or isolated because of anxiety, it can help to know that these are natural feelings that will resolve as your anxiety is relieved.

If you are feeling alone or isolated because of anxiety, it can help to know that these are natural feelings that will resolve as your anxiety is relieved. The important thing is to get help for the underlying problem that's giving you pain and making it hard for you to relax and enjoy other people. Psychotherapy and antidepressants (herbal or conventional) can help. Kava may also help you feel more relaxed and sociable. However, do not combine kava with other medications without professional guidance. (For a detailed explanation of risks involved in taking kava, see chapter 7.)

Weight Gain or Weight Loss

Food is one of the necessities of life, as are air and water. However, it's much more than that. It's also a rich source of comfort, pleasure, and religious and social meaning. Food is wrapped up in many of our most cherished traditions. It's no surprise, then, that food can play a powerful emotional role in our daily lives.

Some people eat too much when they're upset. Others find food distasteful or even sickening when they're anxious. Weight gain and loss can result from emotionally driven changes in eating patterns. The eating disorders anorexia nervosa and bulimia are extreme manifestations of anxiety disrupting a healthful diet.

Proper nutrition is especially important for people suffering from anxiety. A good diet can give us vitality and energy to handle life's many stresses.

It's important to remember that weight gain or loss due to anxiety are symptoms. People tend to focus on their weight as an additional cause of anxiety. However, crash diets aren't going to help restore balance to a mind and body that are struggling to deal with anxiety or depression. Many diet pills on the market have an unfortunate side effect—they tend to have a "speedy" effect that makes anxiety worse. The best approach to unwanted weight loss or gain is to calmly make changes in your life, diet, and, if necessary, medication to address the root cause of the weight change.

Insomnia and Other Sleep Disorders

The best-known sleep disorder is insomnia: the inability to fall asleep or stay asleep. Anxiety, however, can cause not only insomnia but also a whole range of sleep disorders. People suffering from anxiety might go to bed tired and wake up 8 hours later just as tired, wake up too early, or

Dee's Story

Many of us who don't have eating disorders per se still find that our emotional situations can affect our eating patterns. I am reminded of Dee, a woman I met at the gym. Dee was a thin woman who had to eat a lot to maintain the weight she had. Fortunately, she loved to eat. For her, food was the social lubricant in a full and active life, which she lived completely.

However, during times of stress, Dee would stop eating. Food, as she explained, had "simply lost its appeal." She would literally forget to eat, and when she eventually remembered

---

toss and turn relentlessly all night. Sometimes, we "jerk awake" for no reason or sleep much longer than usual. Intense dreaming and nightmares related to anxiety or depression can dramatically interrupt sleep patterns.

Insomnia is one of the most distressing symptoms on our list because lack of sleep makes anxiety even worse and because night offers no relief from the anxiety that has persisted all day long. Naturally, you'll feel worse for wear the next day. And so the cycle continues, often leading to depression if it goes on long enough.

Sleep is very important for health. It is also an area of great sensitivity if we are fearful or anxious. Occasional insomnia, nightmares, and restlessness are normal, even for a healthy individual. None of these situations are cause for alarm unless they persist and disrupt our daily routine.

For many sleep disorders stemming from anxiety, kava may be able to provide relief and leave you fresh and clear the next morning. There is also evidence that the herb va-

that a meal had escaped her, she would decide it was not worth the trouble. In a short time, her weight would start to drop, and so would her energy. Because she was already thin to begin with, the weight loss was unhealthy and physically obvious, which made her feel isolated and drove the vicious cycle.

Dee is now responding well to a self-regulated program of good food, clean water, exercise, fresh air, vitamins, and herbs. Kava is playing a part by helping her get over the rougher bumps in the road of her emotional life.

lerian can be a safe and effective natural aid to sleep. (For a more detailed discussion of insomnia and treatments for it, see chapter 10.)

Other Anxiety Disorders

In its extreme forms, anxiety can lead to more serious symptoms, such as phobias, panic, and obsessions or compulsions. These disorders generally require professional help in the form of therapy, behavior modification, and/or medication.

Phobia Disorder

Phobias are feelings of dread, terror, or panic that are specific to an apparently harmless situation, object, or activity. Phobias can be so strong that they interfere with family life, relationships, and employment. The three types of common phobias are the following:

- *Social phobia,* as in fear of public speaking and "being watched" by other people or extreme reactions to potentially embarrassing situations, such as dropping something in public
- *Simple phobia,* as in extreme fear of specific things or circumstances, such as fear of spiders, fear of driving a car, or fear of flying
- *Agoraphobia* is a fear of being helpless in an unescapable situation (characterized by an avoidance of public places)

Kava is probably not powerful enough to provide significant benefit for these conditions.

Panic Disorder

I previously described the symptoms of a panic attack. Panic attacks can occur in anyone, especially those with anxiety. However, in panic disorder the attacks are recurrent and also more intense. Typically, people suffering from a panic disorder experience symptoms such as shortness of breath, dizziness, faintness, heart palpitations or rapid heartbeat, trembling, sweating, choking, nausea, feelings of unreality, flushes or chills, chest pain, fear of dying, and fear of going crazy. These symptoms intensify during the attack and leave the sufferer exhausted and distraught. Worse, panic attacks are often unrelated to any obvious cause and can wake you from sleep.

Kava is seldom powerful enough to help with such extreme feelings of anxiety. These symptoms generally require professional help, such as behavior modification, therapy, and/or medications.

Obsessive-Compulsive Disorder

Obsessions are unwanted, interfering, repetitious thoughts that cause extreme anxiety. These thoughts or impulses can be extremely unpleasant and include imagined violence or the fear of infection from casual contact with other people. Compulsions are defined as rituals performed in an attempt to reduce anxiety. These behaviors are involuntary, irrational, and repetitious actions meant to ward off catastrophe or discomforting thoughts. However, these rituals have no real connection with the event. Obsessions and compulsions usually appear together and often complement each other.

Obsessive-compulsive problems often respond to antidepressants. Kava is probably not useful for this disorder.

Post-Traumatic Stress Disorder

The result of severe, unusual, and unexpected mental or physical trauma, post-traumatic stress disorder (PTSD) is most often found in veterans of war. However, others, including assault victims and crash survivors, can also suffer from PTSD. People with PTSD regularly re-experience the trauma of the event through nightmares or flashbacks and often suffer from survivor's guilt, emotional numbness, exaggerated startle reaction, anxiety, or depression. Again, kava is probably not strong enough to overcome this serious condition.

The following chapters evaluate the risks and benefits of the leading conventional and alternative therapies for anxiety. If you feel that you exhibit some of the symptoms described in this chapter, the following chapters will help you find a treatment that's appropriate for you.

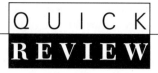

- Anxiety is a fear of the unknown and is a very normal part of life.

- Anxiety can take many forms such as excessive worry, uneasiness and jitters, feeling keyed up and on edge, fear, heart palpitations, chest tightness, "butterflies" in the stomach, headaches, racing thoughts, and more.

- Situational anxieties are usually short term and subside once the "situation" has passed. These anxieties are caused by external sources (outside of the body).

- Anxiety caused by internal sources (inside the body) is more difficult to detect. In fact, people who suffer from inside causes of anxiety might not know why they're anxious, yet the feeling persists.

- Generalized Anxiety Disorder (GAD) is anxiety that has taken on a life of its own, and those who suffer from it should seek professional medical guidance. Kava might be a useful treatment for this condition, as well as more minor feelings of anxiety.

- Kava is probably not effective treatment for severe anxiety-related conditions such as panic disorder, post-traumatic stress disorder or obsessive-compulsive disorder.

What Causes Anxiety?

Anxiety is multidimensional. It has no single cause, just as there is no single pattern to which all anxiety conforms. As we saw in chapter 2, anxiety can be mild or severe, short-term or chronic; it can be triggered by a specific stimulus, or it can be a generalized feeling. Throughout history, there have probably been many causes offered to explain why some people are excessively anxious.

This chapter explains what we know about the causes of anxiety. It will be helpful for understanding how kava works, but if you simply want to find how to take kava, you can skip ahead to chapter 6.

Archaic Theories of Anxiety

In ancient times, those feelings we associate with chronic anxiety were attributed to everything from punishment by gods and devils to being plagued by evil spirits.

Gods and Devils

The earliest humans attributed their strong emotions to divine causes. The gods were considered responsible for all human happiness and suffering. Fear, for example, might be a warning from the gods; sadness and guilt might be the gods' punishment. The Greek god Pan, for in-stance, was thought to fill people with panic when he chose to. In fact, that's where we get the word *panic*.

> **The earliest humans attributed their strong emotions to divine causes. The gods were considered responsible for all human happiness and suffering.**

The "treatment" for such uncomfortable feelings might include sacrifices to appease the gods, consultation with an oracle, or a radical change in lifestyle. These methods were often successful because of the strong belief and practical advice that went along with them. The ancients also had their own herbs and potions, developed over centuries of trial and error, that were usually considered as gifts from the gods. As I explained in chapter 1, kava was perceived by the ancients as a divine herb and was widely used for both its spiritual and its medicinal properties.

The Four Humors

The ancient Greeks believed that gods influenced human emotion and health. They also developed a school of medicine founded on the theory of humors, which was based on close observation of the human body as well as behavior. According to Hippocrates, who helped develop the theory, four liquid "humors" were constantly flowing throughout the body. He named them *blood, phlegm, choler* (yellow bile), and *black bile.* Ill health resulted from an imbalance in the humors. According to this theory, emotions and physical health were all part of the same picture. Too much of any one humor could cause emotional as well as physical disorder. The theory identified four basic human emotional temperaments, corresponding to the four humors: *sanguine* (emotional, happy), related to blood; *phlegmatic* (slow to respond), related to phlegm; *choleric* (angry), related to yellow bile; and *melancholic* (sad), related to black bile. Treatment in this system aimed to restore the balance of the humors. For example, doctors would place leeches on a patient to remove "heat in the blood"—a treatment that was still used in the nineteenth century. The theory of humors dominated Western medicine in the Middle Ages and remained influential long after.

Spiritual Forces

The Christian church was the dominant force in European society during the Middle Ages. Anxiety, depression, and similar conditions were seen as visitations by evil spirits that plagued people who had sinned. Common treatments involved prayer, fasting, local herbal remedies, and, in the worst cases, exorcism. People who suffered from such painful feelings were often blamed for their condition. Spiritual "ills," such as a lack of faith or unatoned sin, were seen as the agents that caused people to feel anxious or depressed. These beliefs had an unfortunate tendency to cause sufferers to be ostracized and mistreated. Even today, traces of such "blame the victim" ideas can be found.

Modern Behavioral Theories

In 1908, the first International Congress of Psycho-Analysis was held in Salzburg, Switzerland, heralding a revolutionary new approach to treating anxiety. Sigmund Freud and his colleagues changed the way in which Western civilization looked at psychic suffering. Instead of blaming the victim or divine or spiritual causes, Freud believed that many kinds of suffering were caused by conflicts that could be understood and resolved. A person's life history might provide clues to her feelings; so might her dreams or other signs of what Freud called the "unconscious" part of the psyche. In other words, Freud saw anxiety not as a force or divine punishment but as a symptom of another, deeper conflict between the individual's desires and guilt or between the individual and another person.

> **The theory of psychoanalysis states that, once the conflicts are identified and resolved through understanding, the painful symptoms will go away.**

His treatment, known as psychoanalysis, encouraged the victim to resolve the inner turmoil by talking about it with a skilled therapist and thus bringing the buried conflicts to light. The theory of psychoanalysis states that, once the conflicts are identified and resolved through understanding, the painful symptoms will go away. An important next step in the understanding and treatment of anxiety, psychoanalysis seems to help many whose conditions before had been deemed hopeless.

Freud's work laid the foundation for psychodynamic theory, which says that anxiety develops from unconscious tension between desires and guilt. In the decades after Freud, several variations on the psychoanalytic model have been developed. Learning theory traces anxiety to traumatic experiences during childhood and aims to help people "unlearn" the fear response they learned as children. Cognitive psychology emphasizes the importance of "self-talk," or the internal dialogue (both good and bad) that constantly goes on within a person's mind. This school of psychology often uses deliberately positive statements, or affirmations, to influence self-talk. Social psychology looks at the effects of poverty, family instability, and other social factors on an individual's mental health.

Until recently, the psychological approach dominated the diagnosis and treatment of anxiety. However, this approach has its limitations—it's only part of the story. As science and medicine became more sophisticated, the physical aspects of anxiety came into perspective to help complete the picture. The chemical makeup of our brains helps explain even more completely the forces that affect feelings of anxiety.

As science and medicine became more sophisticated, the physical aspects of anxiety came into perspective to help complete the picture.

Brain Chemistry

Although much progress has been made using the many psychological techniques, recent research points to brain chemistry as a possible starting point to understanding these disorders. Specific neurotransmitters are used by the brain as signals between cells. The body makes neurotransmitters as needed and then eliminates them when their job is done.

Research has found that neurotransmitters are intricately linked to our emotional states. We're not sure exactly how, but neurotransmitters seem to play a key role in mood disorders, such as depression and anxiety. Changing the levels of certain neurotransmitters within the brain can change our moods, including our feelings of anxiety or depression. These discoveries have opened the way to a whole new approach to treating anxiety. Psychological therapies are very effective for some people with certain conditions, but they can take years of hard work, and they don't work for everyone. Biochemistry is looked on by many in the hope of a simpler treatment—specifically, a pill—that could work faster for a wider range of people and problems. Pills aren't a panacea, but they do offer a good option for many.

> **Psychological therapies are very effective for some people with certain conditions, but they can take years of hard work, and they don't work for everyone.**

For example, the antidepressant drug Prozac is thought to work by affecting levels of a neurotransmitter named *serotonin.* The antianxiety class of drugs known as benzodiazepines, of which Valium is an example, appears to enhance the action of a different neurotransmitter, called *gamma-amino-butyric acid* (GABA). GABA appears to have a calming effect on the brain; in the simplest of terms, the more GABA, the less anxiety. Current knowledge suggests that GABA works by inhibiting the stimulating effects of other neurotransmitters, such as noradrenaline. Essentially, it prevents our neurons from firing too quickly. When our neurons slow down, the muscles relax, breathing and heart rate slow down, body temperature drops, and anxiety is reduced. Furthermore, when GABA is further processed in the brain, it produces another sedating substance known as *gamma hydroxybutyrate,* which also helps promote relaxation.

Genetics

Can you inherit anxiety? It appears that you can. Careful analysis of the frequency of anxiety within families suggests that genetics plays a role. If a genetic cause of anxiety can be discovered, it might lead to new treatments.

However, it is always possible that children learn to be anxious by imitating an anxious parent, rather than through their DNA. It will take further research, perhaps involving identical twins, to help us understand whether anxiety actually runs in families because of genes or whether shared experience is the cause. As with all other health problems, most probably both are involved.

Benzodiazepine drugs relax you by enhancing the action of GABA, and kava appears to work similarly (chapters 5 and 8 will explain these ideas further). The herb valerian, discussed in more detail in chapter 10, also appears to affect GABA receptors, but the data is less convincing for this herb.

Researchers believe that GABA is not the whole story in anxiety. They theorize that there is another natural substance in the brain that works the opposite way, increasing anxiety. This unidentified substance might be released by the brain during periods when extra vigilance is called for, such as while parenting an infant. Researchers speculate that this hypothetical chemical might sometimes be produced unnecessarily, causing chronic anxiety. However, at present this is quite theoretical.

Finally, experience with a new class of drugs indicates that the neurotransmitter serotonin may also be involved in anxiety. Buspirone (BuSpar) is a relatively new nonaddictive and nonsedating antianxiety drug that affects serotonin rather than GABA. While we normally associate serotonin with depression, it seems that there are various different ways in which serotonin affects mood. Altering some of serotonin's effects may help depression, while altering others may relieve anxiety. In the future, unraveling the complicated biology of serotonin and other neurotransmitters will likely lead to the discovery of more useful antianxiety and antidepressant drugs with fewer side effects.

Which Comes First?

As we've just mentioned, changes in brain chemicals can affect anxiety and depression. However, this does not mean that psychological theories of anxiety are all wrong. It is perfectly possible that childhood trauma and other psychological factors can alter the balance of brain chemicals. Furthermore, psychotherapy might have the effect of restoring normal brain chemistry. It's not an either/or situation. As with many other problems, it's best to tackle anxiety from more than one direction at once.

Changing the levels of certain neurotransmitters within the brain can change our moods, including our feelings of anxiety or depression.

Other Factors

Anxiety and anxiety-like symptoms can also result from more immediate sources. Medical illness, medications, and dietary extremes can cause anxiety. Cardiovascular disorders, neurological problems, hypoglycemia, premenstrual syndrome, menopause, thyroid and other glandular disorders, respiratory problems, and immune system dysfunction can produce anxiety symptoms, as can alcoholism and drug addiction. Prescription and over-the-counter drugs, such as cold medicines, diet pills, asthma medications, steroids, and even some antidepressants, can lead to anxiety for some people. Dietary extremes, such as excess caffeine or caffeine-like products such as guarana and mate, can cause anxiety, as can alcohol in its many forms. Check with your pharmacist or physician if you think you might be experiencing anxiety because of any medications you are taking or because of a medical

Check with your pharmacist or physician if you think you might be experiencing anxiety because of any medications you are taking or because of a medical condition.

ical condition. **Warning:** Do not discontinue any necessary medications without first consulting your physician.

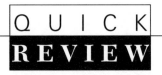

QUICK REVIEW

- It seems most likely that anxiety has many causes. The ancient Greeks ascribed feelings of overwhelming fear, or panic, to the god Pan, and later medical theories tried to make sense of anxiety as an imbalance of humors or as a spiritual illness caused by sin.

- Our modern understanding of anxiety and its causes comes from two main sources: psychology and biochemistry. Psychology sees anxiety as a fundamentally understandable reaction to an internal or external conflict. Biochemistry has advanced to give us clues about the chemical mechanisms in our brains that produce anxiety.

- The neurotransmitter gamma-amino-butyric acid (GABA) appears to be part of the body's natural mechanism for reducing anxiety.

- Benzodiazepine drugs, such as Valium, are thought to increase the action of GABA in the brain. Kava might have a similar effect.

- Anxiety can also be caused by dietary imbalances, a number of physical conditions, alcohol, and certain medications.

- Check with your physician if you think you might be experiencing anxiety because of an illness or a medication.

- Never discontinue any necessary medications without first consulting your physician.

Conventional Treatment for Anxiety

ntianxiety drugs have benefited millions of people in the twentieth century. This chapter evaluates the benefits and risks of the major conventional treatments for anxiety. If you are not interested in this, and simply wish to read about kava, you can skip ahead to the next chapter.

One of the oldest treatments for anxiety is, of course, alcohol. Alcohol profoundly depresses the activity of the brain, including the mechanisms of stress and anxiety. Unfortunately, it also depresses many other brain functions; by the time you've drunk enough to relieve your anxiety, you're partly incapacitated. Also, alcohol is both addictive and toxic to the liver and the brain. When used over a long period of time or to excess, it is a harmful drug with a high personal and social cost.

The mid- and late-1800s brought into use a new sedative medication somewhat less toxic than alcohol but even more addicting: laudanum, an alcoholic mixture of the narcotic drug opium. Laudanum was available without restriction for mere pennies, becoming a best-selling drug in England by the beginning of the 1900s. One of the most popular drugs of the day, laudanum was given for almost every human condition. Because mothers relied on laudanum to comfort crying babies, it was known as "Mother's Quietness" and "Soothing Syrup." Many children died from laudanum overdoses, and many adults became addicted to laudanum before its dangers were understood. Today, tincture of opium is available by prescription only and because of its great addictive potential is used very little.

> **Barbiturates were the dominant anti-anxiety agents pre-scribed during the first half of the twentieth century, until the advent of the benzodiazepine class of drugs.**

Other sedatives discovered in the nineteenth century include paraldehyde, chloral hydrate (when combined with alcohol it's the classic "Mickie Finn" knock-out drops), and bromide salts. However, these new drugs were found to be too toxic or too sedating to be of much general use as antianxiety agents. Paraldehyde is sometimes used today for people undergoing severe alcohol withdrawal symptoms. Chloral hydrate is a prescription sleeping pill and is still used occasionally today as a sedative for infants (this use attests to its relative safety). The bromide salts have fallen into disuse because of their toxicity. As we'll see in this chapter, today's medications for anxiety cause fewer side effects and little to no damage to the body, although addiction is still an issue with many of them.

Barbiturates were discovered in the early 1900s. The original members of this class of drugs were phenobarbital (discovered in 1912) and barbital (discovered in 1913). Many others have followed. Like alcohol, barbiturates suppress the central nervous system (CNS), but they have fewer toxic effects on the rest of the body. Barbiturates reduce anxiety, induce sleep, and prevent epileptic seizures while producing less intoxication than alcohol (when used properly). Barbiturates were the dominant antianxiety agents prescribed during the first half of the twentieth century, until the advent of the benzodiazepine class of drugs (which we will discuss shortly).

> **Since their discovery, the benzodiazepines have dominated conventional treatment for anxiety.**

Unfortunately, barbiturates have many flaws. First, like alcohol and laudanum, they are addictive (and are widely abused as illegal drugs). Also like alcohol, they suppress a number of brain functions all at once. People taking barbiturates during the day often experience "daytime sedation," or drowsiness. Another risk inherent in using barbiturates is that, when taken in high doses or combined with alcohol or other sedatives, they can cause most of the brain to shut down, even turning off the breathing and gag reflex and eventually stopping the heart. Also, because barbiturates nonselectively suppress so many brain functions, they have a tendency to induce tolerance, physical dependence, and potentially lethal reactions during withdrawal.

By the 1950s, the medical community had become concerned about the risks of barbiturates as antianxiety drugs. The search for safer agents led to the discovery of the meprobamate drugs, such as Equanil and Miltown. Somewhat superior to barbiturates, they initially enjoyed popularity as daytime sedatives and sleep aids. However, the meprobamate drugs, like the barbiturates, also caused excessive sedation, physical dependence, and severe intoxication on overdosage.

A real breakthrough came in the late 1950s with the discovery of the drug chlordiazepoxide (Librium) and other drugs of the benzodiazepine group. These drugs, which now include Valium, Xanax, Ativan, and many others, are presently the most common medications used for the treatment of anxiety. Their great advantage is that they are much more specific in action: When used properly, they can reduce anxiety without greatly suppressing other brain activity. They are much less toxic than barbiturates or meprobamate and, when taken in excess, rarely cause a person to stop breathing and die. Since their discovery, this class of drugs has dominated conventional treatment for anxiety.

Benzodiazepines: A Closer Look

The benzodiazepines have come to dominate the antianxiety drug market and in fact represent 5% of all prescriptions written today.

The discovery of benzodiazepines as a new class of antianxiety agents led to the synthesis of over three thousand benzodiazepines, of which some fifty are still clinically used. The most commonly prescribed include chlordiazepoxide (Librium), diazepam (Valium), oxazepam (Serax), clorazepate (Tranxene), lorazepam (Ativan), prazepam (Centrax), alprazolam (Xanax), halazepam (Paxipam), and clonazepam (Klonopin).

These drugs are remarkably effective at reducing anxiety without making a person feel sedated. "Life's problems just don't agitate me so much anymore," said one of my customers who had just been given a prescription for Xanax. "I just handle them; and more importantly, I feel like my normal self." Actually, benzodiazepines are depressants, and they do have a sedative effect in high doses. However, the depressant effect is much more subtle than it is with barbiturates or other, earlier drugs.

How Do We Measure the Effectiveness of an Antianxiety Drug?

Before we look at the effectiveness of the benzodiazepines, we need to take a moment to understand how scientists determine the effectiveness of a medication used to treat anxiety. The major tool used is a set of questions called the Hamilton Anxiety (HAM-A) scale, which is used to rate the overall level of anxiety. The HAM-A scale assigns numbers to a variety of symptoms of anxiety, both mental and physical. Mental anxiety is scored by rating such things as fears and worries; feelings of tension, irritability, nervousness, and restlessness; poor memory; and lack of concentration. Somatic anxiety measures what's happening in the body because of anxiety, such as heart palpitations, stomach discomfort, dizziness, aches, sweating, twitching, and chest pain.

> **The benzodiazepines are remarkably effective at reducing anxiety without making a person feel sedated.**

As you can see by the nature of the questions, the ratings given are largely subjective. You probably mentally rated yourself as you were reading chapter 2 with a quick yes or no. The HAM-A scale assigns a number for each symptom from 0 to 4, with 0 indicating no symptom and 4 indicating severe and incapacitating symptoms. The higher your score, the more anxious you are.

The HAM-A interview, and others like it, is widely used in clinical studies evaluating the effectiveness of antianxiety drugs. In a typical clinical trial, some patients are given placebo treatment, and others are given a real drug. The HAM-A test is given at the beginning and at intervals throughout the trial. The resulting numbers are compared to evaluate the relative effectiveness of the drug versus placebo.

Unfortunately, although the HAM-A is much more reliable than simply asking physicians to decide for themselves whether patients are improving, the scale leaves a lot to be desired. Perhaps the largest problem is that a lot of subjectivity is involved. When different physicians administer the HAM-A interview to the same patient, they might come up with different results. Also, it is not a very sensitive test. Unlike blood pressure measurements, which can detect very fine differences, one person might feel a lot more anxious than another, but both might end up with the same score simply because of how the patients interpret the HAM-A questions and how the clinician observes each patient. Still, the HAM-A scale is the best we have, and if a medication significantly reduces scores, we can take that as a strong indication that the medication is effective.

The HAM-A interview, and others like it, is widely used in clinical studies evaluating the effectiveness of antianxiety drugs.

One final issue arises when determining the effectiveness of benzodiazepines or, indeed, any drug. It's essential to use what's called a double-blind study, in which neither the doctors nor the patients know who has been administered the drug and who has been administered placebo.

In other words, both the doctors and the patients are kept "blind" to prevent the power of suggestion from influencing results. Without this "blinding," the power of suggestion will certainly creep in, and powerfully bias the results (see sidebar, The Power of Placebo).

The Power of Placebo

Just how powerful is placebo treatment? Much more powerful than most people know. In most studies, up to 30% of people show dramatic improvement with placebo pills. For certain illnesses this reaches as high as 70%, and the "benefits" may continue to be felt for years!

Placebo pills also cause a high incidence of imaginary side effects. Before medical researchers started to rely on double-blind studies, they were fooled time and time again by the power of suggestion. Today, we realize that in most cases unless there have been double-blind studies, there is no way to know whether a treatment really works. As we will see in the next chapter, kava has been subjected to studies of this type.

What Do Test Results Say for Benzodiazepine Treatment?

Measured against placebo, the benzodiazepines are clearly effective in reducing the anxiety symptoms of generalized anxiety disorder (GAD) more effectively than placebo. In clinical studies, HAM-A scores show a much greater reduction in anxiety in those patients receiving the benzodiazepines than those in the placebo group. I don't think anyone would dispute the fact that benzodiazepines do work, even for very serious anxiety.

How Do Benzodiazepines Work?

Benzodiazepines were discovered in the late 1950s, beginning with the discovery of chlordiazepoxide in 1957. This discovery came about as scientists were looking for new drugs that had more specific effects on the brain than the generalized suppression of function caused by earlier drugs. Chlordiazepoxide was found to produce "taming" in animals without producing stupor or sleep. In other words, it was more *selective* than older drugs. These intriguing findings served as the first indication of its potential use as a better antianxiety medication, providing relaxation without excessive sedation.

> **The more active the GABA (a naturally occurring brain chemical), the more at-ease you feel.**

Probing deeper for explanations, researchers found that benzodiazepines bind to specific receptors in the brain (see the following explanation). Further research found that a naturally occurring brain chemical called gamma-amino-butyric acid (GABA) binds to a nearby area. As you may recall from chapter 3, GABA appears to play a role in inhibiting nerve activity and thus perhaps in reducing alertness, sleeplessness, and other symptoms of anxiety.

On the basis of this discovery, scientists have formulated a GABA-receptor hypothesis to explain why benzodiazepines are effective in reducing anxiety. To explain this theory further, I must first discuss the nature of a receptor site.

A *receptor* is a specific molecular structure designed to receive a certain chemical known as a *ligand*. When the ligand chemical "locks on" to its designated receptor, a cascade of carefully controlled biological changes occurs. Thus for example, GABA binds to a brain cell and "calms it down." The body, however, likes to have ways to exert fine control over all its processes. One way the body does this is by using other ligands that can either interfere with or enhance the ability of a major ligand to do its work. These other ligand chemicals can bind to nearby sites and physically distort the shape of the primary receptor to make it either a better or a worse fit for the ligand. According to the GABA-receptor hypothesis, benzodi-azepines bind to a portion of the GABA receptor and thus make that receptor bind to GABA better. In other words, these drugs act to increase the action of GABA in the brain, and the more active the GABA, the more at-ease you feel. In essence, the benzodiazepines make cells listen when GABA talks.

This effect is much more specific than that exerted by other sedatives and allows benzodiazepines to reduce anxiety without producing too many side effects. Interestingly, kava appears to work by interacting with GABA as well, although probably not in the same way. (This is discussed further in chapter 5.)

Benefits and Drawbacks of Benzodiazepines

Compared with all the previous conventional antianxiety medications, benzodiazepines are effective and much safer. Before benzodiazepines came onto the scene, it was easy to overdose to the point of death with meprobamate and the barbiturates. These drugs nonselectively depressed the CNS more and more with increasing doses, progressing from calming to drowsiness, sleep, unconsciousness, coma, and finally to fatal depression of breathing and the heart. However, even with high doses of benzodiazepines alone, it is virtually impossible to cause fatal CNS depression.

Nonetheless, benzodiazepines are far from perfect. Their major drawback is that they're habit-forming. In a sense, this is because they work so well—people with anxiety simply don't want to contemplate going without their medication. Whenever an anxiety-provoking event or thought occurs, people taking benzodiazepines might want to turn toward the drug and not try to fight the anxiety any other way. "I loved taking Xanax—it made me feel great, happy—but then I began to worry that I'd have to take it for the rest of my life," said Joan. This is a problem because benzodiazepines don't cure anxiety. Their benefits don't carry over once you stop taking them. In fact, when some benzodiazepines are abruptly discontinued, one can experience an unpleasant phenomenon called "rebound anxiety." Some people find that their own natural ability to deal with anxiety diminishes while they're taking the drug. Joan went on to add, "I tried tapering off Xanax once, after I'd been taking it for about 18 months. Wow, did I feel raw and helpless! My feelings and my life's problems were staring me right in the face, and I had no coping skills to handle them. I went . . . no, I *ran* straight back to my doctor's office. I didn't know where else to turn."

Benzodiazepines are far from perfect. Their major drawback is that they're habit forming.

One can say that it is no different with other diseases. Depressed people might find it scary to contemplate quitting Prozac as well, but there is a difference: Benzodiazepines give almost immediate results, whereas Prozac and other antidepressants take 3 to 6 weeks to work. It's hard to become addicted to something that takes a month to do anything. The instant gratification of benzodiazepines allows more of an addictive pattern to develop.

In addition, the body becomes accustomed to having the benzodiazepines around and starts to need them. Benzodiazepines are physically addicting, and sudden discontinuation can lead to severe and even fatal withdrawal symptoms. A tolerance can also develop to benzodiazepines, leading some people to progressively increase their dose. However, this latter problem doesn't occur as often as previously thought and is generally limited to people with a history of addiction to other drugs.

It seems to be human nature to overindulge and even to abuse substances that alter our moods and give us some relief from the harshness of life. Because of this, benzodiazepines have at times become the victim of their own success. They make people feel so good that they have been used illegally as a recreational drug, either by themselves or mixed with alcohol or other drugs.

Benzodiazepines were also greatly overprescribed: In the 1960s, they became known as "Mommy's little helpers" when they were given to women fairly indiscriminately by physicians.

Side Effects

After their heyday of indiscriminate use in the 1960s and 1970s, benzodiazepines fell into disfavor for a time. However, they have been reappraised in recent years. Many physicians have found them to be quite useful, especially for treating anxiety and sleeplessness. Because the tendency to increase the dose is not as great as previously thought, physicians are no longer so afraid of using them in the long term or in high doses if necessary. With careful supervision, many people can take them for a long time without needing to increase the dosage.

Benzodiazepines also have a few other potential side effects, including mild feelings of sedation, impaired body movements, confusion, dizziness, headache, weight gain, menstrual irregularities, and increased incidence of osteoporosis (probably due to prolonged inactivity).

Warning: When benzodiazepines are taken for long periods of time and then abruptly withdrawn, severe withdrawal symptoms, including seizures, can occur. You should never stop taking benzodiazepines except under the supervision of a physician.

Check with your physician if you have concerns about possible side effects from any antianxiety medications that you're taking or thinking of taking. Different benzodiazepines

Prescription Medications for Severe Anxiety

For people who suffer from severe anxiety, prescription medications can offer relief and hope. As a pharmacist, I know this from the many stories I've heard from customers. One physician friend commented, "Among my patients, I think I've noticed that Xanax in particular is highly specific for anxiety and is nearly side-effect free. I know people who've been on it for years without escalating the dosage."

have different side effects. If one medication doesn't work for you, you and your physician can explore others.

Buspirone

A relatively new class of drugs for the treatment of anxiety is buspirone, which has been marketed since 1986 as BuSpar. Buspirone was discovered by researchers who were trying to develop an antipsychotic drug. Although buspirone proved not to have any antipsychotic properties, it was found to be effective in reducing anxiety. "When my doctor switched me from Xanax to BuSpar, I felt remarkably better," remarked Hal, a busy business executive. "My anxiety was relieved, my tension headaches gone, and my work productivity improved. I'm less sluggish on this stuff, and my doctor is less worried about me taking it for a longer time."

Buspirone has several advantages compared with the benzodiazepines. Most important, buspirone is nonaddictive. Unlike the benzodiazepines, buspirone isn't a sedative and usually doesn't cause drowsiness or mental impairment. Also, buspirone works slowly, requiring weeks to reach its full effect. (In this respect, it is like kava.) While this makes it less useful for instant relief, it has the advantage of making buspirone less psychologically addictive.

Today, buspirone is becoming a well-established alternative to benzodiazepines, especially for people who need to maintain daytime alertness or are reluctant to risk becoming addicted to a medication. It is used to manage anxiety disorders and provide short-term relief of anxiety and is especially beneficial to those with generalized anxiety of limited severity.

Buspirone has several advantages compared with the benzodiazepines. Most important, buspirone is nonaddictive.

Buspirone is beneficial to both psychic (mood, behavior, and intellectual symptoms) and somatic (muscular, sensory, cardiovascular, gastrointestinal, and autonomic effects) symptoms of anxiety. It acts differently from other antianxiety agents in that it is not a sedative at all. It is not chemically or pharmacologically related to the benzodiazepines, barbiturates, or other sedative or antianxiety agents.

Scientists don't actually know how buspirone works. It seems to have a selective affinity for certain serotonin receptors but not for others. Serotonin is a chemical found in many parts of the body, including the CNS, where it acts as a central neurotransmitter. Serotonin seems to be implicated in our moods, but, contrary to what you might read, we don't know exactly how it works. Buspirone also affects other neurotransmitters, such as norepinephrine and dopamine. The bottom line is that we have only vague clues as to the action of buspirone, so "we just don't know" is the only honest reply to "how does buspirone work?" Further research is needed before we'll understand buspirone's effects completely.

Buspirone has not been shown to be as helpful for panic attacks as the more powerful benzodiazepines (or certain antidepressants). It is also not as effective by itself as a treatment for obsessive-compulsive disorders as are some of the antidepressants. People who respond well to benzodiazepines might not find buspirone as effective. We don't yet understand why some drugs work for certain types of anxiety but not for others. Much has yet to be learned about exactly how buspirone works, on which kinds of anxiety it's most effective, and how it might work in combination with other drugs to produce desired results. It will take a long time for scientists to understand the exact nature of our brain chemistry and how it affects the many kinds of anxiety, and it might take just as long to understand how drugs and herbs act in our brains.

The high cost of buspirone remains an issue for those without good health insurance.

Although buspirone is not a true sedative, some people (approximately 10%) do feel drowsy when taking it. Because it can cause drowsiness, caution is advised when driving or operating machinery. Dizziness, headaches, and other side effects can occur in about 5 to 10% of patients.

Buspirone is an increasingly popular treatment for many people suffering from anxiety. It makes a good alternative to the benzodiazepines because it is relatively safe, nonaddictive, and generally free of sedative effects. However, buspirone isn't effective for panic attacks or for severe anxiety disorders, such as obsessive-compulsive disorder. For many people, the quick-acting, more potent benzodiazepines are more effective than buspirone, especially for those who are already on benzodiazepines. The high cost of buspirone also remains an issue for those without good health insurance because nearly all benzodiazepines are available in the form of their far less expensive generic counterparts.

Other Antianxiety Medications

As we learned in chapter 2, anxiety can be rooted in depression. One widely used therapeutic approach for depression-related anxiety is to treat the primary cause—the depression. The leading class of drugs used to treat depression today are the selective serotonin reuptake inhibitors (SSRIs), the best known of which is Prozac. SSRIs act to increase the levels of serotonin in the brain, and this

is thought to explain their antidepressant effects. For reasons that are not entirely clear, most antidepressants can also relieve anxiety. The effect takes several weeks to develop. Unfortunately, the initial side effects of some antidepressants can actually increase a sense of anxiety, so have some patience. Antidepressants are nonaddictive, and the newer ones are relatively safe and have few side effects. (For a more detailed discussion of antidepressants, see *The Natural Pharmacist Guide to St. John's Wort and Depression.*)

One widely used therapeutic approach for depression-related anxiety is to treat the primary cause—the depression.

Finally, a class of drugs called beta-blockers, such as propranolol (Inderal), can reduce body symptoms associated with specific situational anxieties (such as giving a speech before a room full of people) and phobias. These drugs slow the heart rate and therefore help relieve the racing-heart feeling associated with certain anxieties.

Beyond Drugs

Medications are not the only approach to treating anxiety. Modern treatment of anxiety has evolved along two paths: medication and psychotherapy. Interestingly, the reason that medication is currently the leading edge of treatment might be because it is better adapted to deal with the nature of our overly anxious society. What do I mean by this? Medication is quick and simple compared to psychotherapy, which takes time, patience, and personal commitment. If the fast pace of modern life is one of the factors that makes us anxious, it also urges us to look for quick fixes for our anxiety. Most medical doctors are accustomed to prescribing medications for whatever ails us, and patients are accustomed to demanding medications from their physicians.

However, for some types of anxiety disorder, such as phobias, psychotherapy is still the preferred treatment, because drugs are not very effective for these conditions. A therapist can often help a person "get used to" the thing or situation that the person fears. Because the fear-inducing thing or situation might not be encountered every day, taking a daily antianxiety agent is usually not necessary.

Psychotherapy has two other advantages over drugs: It gives you coping skills for a lifetime, and it benefits your life in general. A good customer, and a very private woman named Doris, exclaimed, "I always took the strong, stoic approach to my life's problems. But when I finally realized I needed help, I began seeing a therapist for the first time in my life. At first it was a little scary thinking about things I used to just power through, but after a while I got to liking it. Now I can say that not only did I learn how to solve the problems that created my initial anxiety, but by looking at my life as a whole, I was able to work through other uncomfortable issues, too. I'm a happier, more open, and relaxed person today than I ever was in my whole life. Why didn't I do this sooner?"

As a pharmacist, I often suggest to my customers that if they feel that they need more than what their medication is offering or if it isn't doing the trick, they should consider therapy. I generally recommend that they continue to take their medication while they're finding and settling into a therapy that's right for them. Then, after therapy has started, any medication changes can be made by the physician at the appropriate time.

There are other alternatives to conventional treatment besides psychotherapy. The remainder of this book examines the benefits, risks, and effectiveness of a natural medication for anxiety: kava. Chapter 9 discusses other herbal and alternative treatments that might be useful as well.

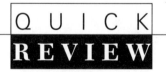

QUICK REVIEW

- Modern antianxiety drugs offer effective relief with relatively few side effects.
- Benzodiazepines, such as Valium and Xanax, are by far the most widely prescribed antianxiety medications available today. They work by affecting the neurotransmitter gamma amino-butyric acid (GABA).
- Kava also appears to affect GABA.
- Benzodiazepines can cause sedation, tolerance, addiction, and serious symptoms of withdrawal.

- Never stop taking benzodiazepines except under the supervision of a physician.
- Another widely used modern antianxiety medication is buspirone, which has fewer side effects than the benzodiazepines and no risk of dependency or sedation.
- Buspirone is not as fast acting or as strong as the benzodiazepines, so it is not useful for those needing immediate pronounced anxiety relief.
- Selective serotonin reuptake inhibitors (SSRIs), such as Prozac, or other antidepressants can relieve anxiety as well.
- Beta-blockers are heart medications used for situational anxieties, such as that experienced when giving a speech.
- Psychotherapy is another tool that can be useful in treating anxiety. It gives people lasting benefits that belong to them. Psychotherapy often works well in conjunction with medication and other therapies.

Kava

The Scientific Evidence

In the United States, herbs have only recently begun to be taken seriously by conventional medicine. However, in Germany and other European nations, the situation is different. Herbs are much more commonly prescribed in Europe and are frequently the subject of objective scientific inquiry. In addition, this research is done on herbal products that are manufactured under pharmaceutical industry standards. For this reason, all of the serious scientific evidence for kava comes from European trials.

Older studies focused on the kavalactones, the main chemical constituents of kava. However, more recent studies have evaluated the effectiveness of whole kava, comparing it to either placebo treatment or conventional medications. Chapter 8 discusses the research that compares kava to standard antianxiety treatments. This chapter looks at the placebo trials, which form the most important scientific basis for using kava as a treatment for anxiety.

What Research Says About Kava's Effectiveness

Four double-blind placebo-controlled studies have been conducted on the effectiveness of kava in treating anxiety, enrolling about 240 participants.[1-4] In addition, several placebo-controlled studies have been conducted on kavalactones extracted from kava. Taken together, the evidence strongly indicates that kava is an effective treatment for many symptoms of anxiety.

HAM-A and CGI Rating Scales

Before we look at the research, we need to examine the two major anxiety testing scales used in these studies: the Hamilton Anxiety (HAM-A) scale introduced in chapter 4 and the Clinical Global Impressions (CGI) scale. The HAM-A is used to rate generalized anxiety. It measures overall anxiety symptoms of both mental anxiety and somatic anxiety. As mentioned in chapter 4, mental anxiety includes anxious mood, insomnia, depression, worry, and fear. Somatic anxiety refers to internal physical symptoms, such as sweating, muscle tension, increased heart rate, shallow breathing, queasiness in the stomach, urgency to urinate, and trembling. The HAM-A rating scale uses a system that assigns a number from 0 to 4 for each symptom, with 0 indicating no symptom and 4 indicating a very severe and incapacitating symptom. The higher the total score, the more serious the anxiety. A person with no anxiety would have a score of 0, but probably no living, breathing person would rate this low!

Researchers use the HAM-A scale before and after treatment to measure any difference in symptoms that might have been changed due to the treatment. They also use another measurement tool: the CGI scale. Rather than focusing on particular "symptoms," this scale attempts to determine how the person feels overall. One must experience a relatively greater improvement to be noticed on the CGI scale than on the HAM-A scale—enough of an improvement to make a real difference in a person's life.

The Volz Study

This study stands out among all of the research conducted on kava. The German Volz study enrolled 101 individuals with anxiety symptoms and followed them for 6 months.[5] The study was conducted according to modern research standards, using an especially rigorous mathematical analysis called "intention to treat," and involved enough people for the results to be meaningful.

Ten medical centers participated in this study. Each participant suffered from at least one of five anxiety-related illnesses: generalized anxiety disorder, agoraphobia (fear of open spaces), specific phobia (a more particular fear), social phobia (fear of being among people), and adjustment disorder with anxiety (anxiety caused by a difficult life situation). These diagnoses were determined by a standard method of identifying psychiatric illnesses, the *DSM-III-R (Diagnostic and Statistical Manual of Mental Disorders)*.

The HAM-A is a scale used to rate generalized anxiety. The higher the score, the more serious the anxiety.

For 1 week, all participants were given placebo treatment, then half were given 300 mg of a standardized 70% kavalactone extract daily for 24 weeks. (For a discussion of standardized extracts of kava, see chapter 6.) The remainder stayed on placebo, and neither doctors nor participants knew which treatment was which.

A minimum HAM-A score of at least 19 was required to participate in this study. This score indicates a significant level of anxiety (remember: the higher the score, the more severe the anxiety), but the average HAM-A score of participants was even higher—about 31. Over the course of the study, the test subjects were evaluated at 4-week intervals using the HAM-A scale to see how much their anxiety improved. The CGI test was also administered, but not as frequently—at the beginning of the study and then again at 12 weeks and 24 weeks.

Interestingly, both kava and placebo treatment significantly reduced anxiety levels. (The power of placebo never fails to astonish!) At week 4, both groups had improved significantly and by about the same amount. The average HAM-A score was now only about 24. However, by week 8, the kava group had pulled ahead. Average HAM-A scores were only 17 as compared to 20 in the placebo group. Over the remaining weeks of the study, both groups improved, but kava increased its lead. At the end of the study, those taking kava had improved their HAM-A scores by almost 70%. Those taking placebo also gradually improved, but at the end of the study they had plateaued at a 50% improvement. The difference between the two groups was mathematically significant from week 8 on.

The CGI scores also showed that kava was more effective than placebo. At the end of the 25 weeks, physicians rated 69% of the participants taking kava as "much improved," compared to only 37% of those on placebo (see figure 2).

This study shows two things quite clearly. First, placebo treatment is remarkably effective at reducing anxiety symptoms. This reminds us of the need for double-blind trials such as this one. If no placebo group had been used, kava might have seemed to be impressively beneficial even if it didn't work at all.

Second, because a placebo group was used, this study provides strong evidence that kava does have some effect

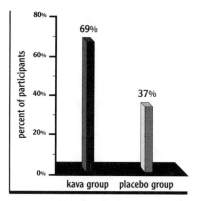

Figure 2. *Percent of participants rated "much improved" (based on CGI scores) after 24 weeks of kava in double-blind study* (Volz, 1997)

of its own apart from the power of suggestion. It appears safe to conclude from this study that kava is an effective treatment for anxiety.

However, few studies are perfect. This one had one drawback at least: It included participants with different forms of anxiety. Thus, this study can't tell us which types of anxiety kava is best for. Nonetheless, this is the best study on kava performed so far, and by itself it gives strong evidence that this herb is an effective treatment for anxiety.

Other Double-Blind Studies of Whole Kava

Other double-blind studies have been conducted on kava, and all have found kava to be effective as well. Interestingly, in these studies the results showed up much more quickly, in just 1 week. For example, a double-blind placebo-controlled study followed 40 women with menopause-related anxiety symptoms, with average HAM-A scores about the same as those in the study just mentioned.[6] The treatment group in this study was again given 300 mg of a 70% kavalactone extract daily. In this case, by week 1, the HAM-A scores of the group receiving kava decreased by 50%, compared to a much smaller improvement in the placebo group. At 4 weeks, the improvement in scores was nearly 80%. By contrast, placebo treatment never produced more than a 30% improvement in scores. The CGI scale of over-all improvement also found a comparatively better result with kava than placebo.

Similar results were seen in another study of 40 women with menopause-related anxiety symptoms.[7]

In some studies, kava worked in 1 week, but in another the effects weren't apparent until it had been taken for 2 months.

Based on the results of these two studies, kava is specifically recommended as an herb useful for women going through meno-pause. (For information on other natural treatments for meno-pause, see *The Natural Pharma-cist Guide to Menopause.*)

It's not just menopause re-lated anxiety that can respond to kava in a week. A study that in-volved a wide variety of anxiety also found an effect within 1 week. In this double-blind trial, 58 individuals with average HAM-A scores of about 25 were given either kava (300 mg of a 70% kavalactone extract daily) or placebo for a period of 4 weeks.[8,9] Within 1 week, the treatment group began to show better results than the placebo group, and the differ-ence increased during the course of the study.

The bottom line is that although kava does appear to be effective for anxiety, we don't know exactly how much time it takes to work. More studies, especially ones that focus on specific types of anxiety, need to be performed to fully clarify this issue.

Study on an Herbal Mixture Containing Kava

One double-blind placebo-controlled study on kava has been conducted in the United States. This study evaluated the effectiveness of a commercial herb mixture containing kava in 60 people with mild anxiety that was generally consistent with the hassles of daily life.[10] The mixture also included other herbs that are thought to have relaxing effects, including passionflower, chamomile, hops, and schisandra.

Instead of using the HAM-A test, researchers used a variety of less-well-known scales that measure the stress of everyday life. The results showed good results with the kava mixture but no effect at all with placebo.

However, this study has many problems. The lack of any placebo response at all is highly unusual (almost unheard of) for studies of stress and mild anxiety. Some benefit should have been seen. In addition, because the mixture did not contain kava

Based on the results of these two studies, kava is specifically recommended as an herb useful for women going through menopause.

alone, the extent to which the results were due to kava itself is not clear. Finally, the results of this study have not been published in a scientific journal. For all these reasons, this study is considerably less trustworthy than the others described earlier.

Lucy's Story

Lucy took medications from time to time when her anxiety levels peaked, but she didn't like taking them. "They work, but I couldn't get anything done while I was taking them. They slow me down!" she complained.

One day when she came into the store, I recommended that she try kava. I wasn't surprised when Lucy phoned the next afternoon, complaining that the kava didn't work, that it was just "money down the drain and a waste of time." If I could get her to slow down enough to hear me, I thought I might just have a chance to help her understand the nature of how kava works. After I repeated myself three times, she finally seemed

Research on Kavalactones

In all the studies just described, researchers used concentrated extracts of whole kava root, containing many ingredients mixed together. However, earlier research from the 1960s and 1970s focused on one constituent of kava, called *kavain* (or *kawain*). Kavain is believed to be one of the main active ingredients in kava and, according to the results of seven double-blind placebo-controlled studies, is an effective treatment for anxiety.[11] However, keep in mind that the kavain used in this research is a special concentrated product that is not identical to ordinary kava extract.

Theories About How Kava Works

As we saw in chapter 1, the active constituents of kava appear to be the kavalactones (one of which is kavain), a group of chemicals with antianxiety, sedative, muscle-to hear what I was telling her. "It's not instantaneous like Valium," I said, and at last she understood.

It took Lucy almost 1 month to get the full benefits from kava, but by then she was a true believer. I overheard her chatting with her neighbor in the aisle, extolling the virtues of kava. "It's gentle, yet effective . . . but you gotta give it time. Its effects worked on me slowly, but I was able to get all my work done and take care of my family, too." Then she laughed. "I sound like a walking commercial for this stuff!" Of course, anecdotes like this one don't prove that kava is effective. For that you need research, such as the studies described in this chapter.

relaxant, and analgesic properties.[12] These substances seem to affect gamma-amino-butyric acid (GABA).

As we saw in chapter 4, GABA is a brain chemical that appears to produce a naturally calming effect. Benzodiazepine drugs are believed to work by enhancing the ability of GABA to bind to GABA receptors. Early research on kava did not find that it influenced GABA much,[13] but more recent research has found that kavalactones do seem to influence GABA.[14] Apparently, early studies missed this because they were looking in the wrong parts of the brain. Kava seems to produce the greatest effect on GABA in areas of the brain related to emotion and memory. The first studies had examined parts of the brain connected to thought and movement, where kava apparently does not interact with GABA.

In addition, kava doesn't seem to affect GABA in the same way that benzodiazepine drugs do. Whereas benzodiazepines make it easier for GABA to bind to the receptors that already exist, kava appears to work by increasing the number of GABA-binding sites instead. The net effect might be the same: If there are more binding sites, the chance of GABA binding to some of them increases, and it has a greater chance to produce its calming effects.

Kava seems to produce the greatest effect on GABA in areas of the brain related to emotion and memory, not the areas connected to thought and movement.

This study uncovered another interesting fact. When kava is taken with a barbiturate, it heightens (technically, *potentiates*) the barbiturate's effects. This result seems to indicate that both barbiturates and kava work within the same general mechanisms in the nervous system. It also suggests that it might not be safe to combine kava with barbiturates. (For more information on potential interactions between kava and sedating drugs, see chapter 7.)

However, kava might also work in another way. Two recent reports suggest that kavalactones can suppress the release of glutamate, an amino acid neurotransmitter.[15,16] Glutamate works opposite to GABA by stimulating the brain. Perhaps kava works in two ways at once, both increasing the calming effects of GABA and decreasing the stimulating effects of glutamate. Some conventional antiseizure drugs appear to function in much this way, but we still don't know a lot on the subject.

What Doctors Say

The best way to find out how well a medication works is to look at the results of double-blind placebo-controlled studies. Another way is to interview physicians who use it for their patients. Although this isn't a scientifically valid method, it can sometimes give a "flavor" of how a treatment works.

Most physicians interviewed for this book agree that kava shows mild to moderate effectiveness in the treatment of anxiety. One neurologist expressed very positive experiences with kava as a treatment for anxiety. "Quality kava products are quite helpful for the rough periods in people's lives. Kava does what my patients want it to do on two important aspects. One, it takes care of the problem of anxiety. Two, it does so without leaving the person feeling impaired. I'm impressed with its gentle action and lack of side effects."

However, he adds a cautionary note as well. "I think that people with chronic cases of anxiety should see both a physician and therapist. 'Medications' plus 'talk' works best. And I don't recommend taking kava for more than a few months. We don't know enough about its long-term safety."

Some psychotherapists are also recommending that their clients try kava. One prominent psychotherapist says, "I am quite happy to see kava so readily available. I find it a useful treatment when clients first come to see me for an evaluation of their anxiety problems. It can give some quick relief while we are spending in-depth time getting to the root causes of their anxieties."

Because kava heightens the effects of barbiturates, it might not be safe to combine it with such drugs.

However, most physicians and psychotherapists feel that kava is not as powerful as drug treatment. (For a detailed discussion of this point, see chapter 8.) According to Steven Bratman, M.D., "Kava's effects are subtle, it reduces anxiety. Benzodiazepine drugs, on the other hand, shut it off almost entirely."

However, Bratman thinks that for most people, kava is actually better. "Kava's gentler effect is a big advantage. By reducing anxiety, it helps you cope, but because it doesn't completely take anxiety away, it doesn't act so much like a crutch. People taking benzodiazepines often seem to forget the basic ways to deal with anxiety that we all use at times. They don't go for long walks, talk to their friends, take a hot shower, or work in the garden when they feel anxious. They just pop a pill. The drug becomes the total and only solution for anxiety. But because kava is not so totally effective, people who take it still practice ordinary ways of calming down. I think this is much healthier."

Most physicians interviewed for this book agree that kava shows mild to moderate effectiveness in the treatment of anxiety.

Nonetheless, Bratman thinks that in some cases standard antianxiety drugs are necessary. "In extremely severe anxiety, kava probably will not work. It is best used for mild to moderate anxiety."

Some people don't like kava. "While most people find kava to be gentle and mild, others feel unpleasantly drowsy and confused when they take it. All treatments are like that: You have to experiment a little to see what works best for you."

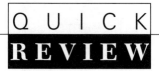

- Good scientific evidence tells us that kava is an effective treatment for anxiety.
- In the largest study, kava took about 8 weeks to reach its full effect in people with various forms of anxiety. Two studies suggest that kava is helpful for menopause-related anxiety, producing benefits within 1 week.
- One of the ingredients of kava, kavain, has also been found to be an effective antianxiety treatment.
- We don't know exactly how kava works. Current research indicates that the kavalactones in kava might work in two ways at once. They appear to increase the number of GABA-binding sites in parts of the brain, helping GABA to keep us calm. They also appear to work on the other side of the problem as well, inhibiting the action of a neurotransmitter, glutamate, that activates the brain.
- Kava should not be combined with other sedative drugs.

How to Take Kava

After reading about the benefits of kava, you might be interested in trying it as a treatment for anxiety. This chapter will tell you what the proper dosage is, where to get it, and what to expect from it. It will also explain certain issues that arise because kava is an herb and not a drug.

Dosage

Kava products are standardized to their content of kava's presumed active ingredients, the kavalactones. (See following discussion for more information on what it means to standardize an herb.) Most products contain either 30 or 70% kavalactones. The bottle should say how many milligrams of kavalactones there are per tablet. (If it doesn't, you can calculate it by from the total milligrams of kava and the percentage of kavalactones.)

To treat anxiety, the usual dose of kava should supply 20 to 70 mg of kavalactones 3 times daily. This is a fairly wide dose range because everyone responds differently. I recommend starting with about 50 mg of kavalactones 3 times daily and then adjusting up or down, depending on the results. If your initial dosage doesn't work well enough, take more; if you start feeling sleepy, take less.

According to German standards, your total intake of kavalactones should not exceed 300 mg daily because at that point you won't be getting any additional benefit but will be more at risk for side effects.[1] Also, German guidelines recommend using kava for only 3 months so as not to become psychologically dependent on it. During that period, it's rec-

To treat anxiety, the usual daily dose of kava should supply 20 to 70 mg of kavalactones 3 times daily.

ommended that you find more permanent ways (such as those described in chapter 9) to cope with your anxiety.

Which Form of Kava Should I Take?

Kava comes in many strengths, depending on kavalactone content, ranging from 30 to 70% concentration. Some people feel that the 30% form actually works better than the 70% form, perhaps because the larger amount of other, unknown ingredients in the 30% form may add to kava's calming effect. In the more highly purified kava products, these other ingredients might be eliminated. Kava comes in different dosage forms as well: capsules and tablets, tinctures and extracts, teas, and even kava drinks. Where to begin?

Kava teas and drinks are probably not the best choice, except for those who really like kava's strong taste and numbing of the mouth. Tinctures concentrate the product so that you can swallow the kava quickly, but there is still a taste that lingers. Pill forms are the most convenient because you won't taste the kava at all.

Kava teas and drinks are probably not the best choice, except for those who really like kava's strong taste and numbing of the mouth.

Kava can be obtained by itself or in combination with other ingredients. Some people like combination products because they are convenient—you can get the benefit of taking several herbs at once without having to buy a lot of bottles. Kava is frequently sold in combination with other relaxing herbs such as valerian, hops, and passionflower, or minerals such as calcium and magnesium. (See chapter 9 for more information on these other natural treatments for anxiety.) However, there has not been any research to tell us whether these treatments work well together. It is also possible that such combinations could be dangerous, although no serious adverse effects have been reported.

Kava is also often sold in combination with the antidepressant herb St. John's wort (see the *Natural Pharmacist Guide to St. John's Wort and Depression* for more information). The idea behind this combination comes from conventional medicine, in which antianxiety medications are often combined with antidepressant drugs. One treatment addresses the anxiety and the other works with the depression that often accompanies or even causes it. However, again we don't know how well kava and St. John's wort work together, and whether it is safe to combine them.

Furthermore, combination products do not give you control over the dosage levels of only one ingredient. For example, if the dosage of kava in one capsule isn't enough for you, and you're thinking of taking two capsules to get the amount of kava you want, you would be taking twice the dosage of everything else in the capsule, which might prove to be too much for you. Combination products don't offer the dosage flexibility that single products offer. I recommend you take individual herbs, and identify the right dose for you before adding others.

How Much Does Kava Cost, and Where Do I Get It?

Kava is popular these days, and it's available wherever herbs are sold—in pharmacies; in health-food, grocery, and mass merchandise stores; and by mail order.

Pill forms of kava are the most convenient because you won't taste the kava at all.

Depending on the form purchased, a typical dosage generally costs from $15 to $25 per month (which falls into the normal range of prices for herbal products). Generally, the least expensive forms of kava are the tinctures and extracts. Teas and drinks might seem cheaper, but they might not deliver an effective therapeutic amount of kava. Tablets and capsules are the most popular and easiest to use forms for most people, so they might be worth the price difference.

What to Expect from Treatment

Kava is most likely to be effective if you suffer from mild to moderate levels of anxiety. If you suffer from frequent panic attacks or severe, debilitating anxiety, this herb probably won't be as effective, and you might need medical assistance.

However, for anxiety that is merely unpleasant, kava can provide adequate relief. Most people report noticeable results in 1 week, but optimum anxiety reduction can take 1 month or more. This means that you might experience a gentle, gradual elimination of many of the symptoms of anxiety (although everyone is different). Be patient. Over time, you might feel more at ease with your life.

> **You don't want kava to become a crutch. It would be better to learn how to stay calm without popping a pill or even an herb.**

Don't forget, however, that kava by itself does not solve anything. If you continue to need kava for more than 3 months, seek medical attention. You need to make sure that you don't suffer from some medical cause of anxiety, such as high thyroid levels. Also, you don't want kava to simply become a crutch. It would be better to learn how to stay calm without popping a pill or even an herb. Remember though, the combination of learning new coping skills along with using a drug or herb can be very helpful.

Some people experience relief with kava fairly rapidly. For this reason, it is worth trying kava for short-term stress-related anxiety. For example, Gene, a pharmacist friend of mine, shared an interesting kava story with me. He was attending a weeklong pharmacy association meeting in New York when, as he told me, "All hell broke loose." To start it off, his luggage didn't arrive with him on the plane, which meant that he was going to have to perform his speaking program in his casual clothes. "No big deal," he thought. That was when he realized that he had left his slides behind on the airport desk while checking on his missing luggage.

Gene lay awake most of the night, trying to figure out an alternative plan for his presentation. He decided to give a show-and-tell type of presentation using actual products plus an overhead projector for factual information. The talk was on herbal medicines, so he headed off in a big rush in the morning to purchase the herbs he needed for his presentation. Frazzled, Gene decided to try some of the kava he bought for his talk. Having never taken it before, he was surprised by the result. "It calmed my mind enough so I had room to think," he said. "Time seemed to slow down, and I sensed I had all the time in the world to prepare. I seemed to forget all about the earlier hassles. I felt refreshed and sharp."

Some people experience relief from kava fairly rapidly. For this reason, it is worth trying kava for short-term stress-related anxiety.

Gene reported that his presentation went well and that he felt no let-down after the kava wore off. In his case, kava worked well for short-term, situational distress.

Quality Issues

When using herbs, a challenge arises that you won't find with medications. Medications always have a measured, quality-assured, and clearly defined strength listed on the package. For example, a bottle of aspirin labeled "325 mg" contains exactly 325 milligrams of the single chemical

Barbara's Story

One customer named Barbara told me, "I've suffered from anxiety for the past several years and have tried many different herbs. I don't like to take drugs, you see." I asked her whether she had tried kava. "Funny you should ask," she replied. "I've been taking it for 2 weeks now, but it isn't doing a thing. I'm in here today trying to decide what to take next." I suggested to Barbara that as long as she had already bought the bottle of kava, she might as well take it a little longer. Two weeks later she excitedly reported, "I still have my ups and downs, but I can cope with them better. They don't seem to bowl me over so much." For Barbara, it wasn't a matter of the wrong herb but a matter of patience.

called aspirin. As a pharmacist, I know that every bottle of 325-mg aspirin contains the same active ingredient, no matter which manufacturer produced it.

However, with herbs the situation is different. Herbs are plants that contain dozens, hundreds, or even thousands of ingredients. Unlike a tablet of aspirin, an herb does not contain only one active compound. Furthermore, the chemical constituents of herbs vary, depending on where and how the herb was grown; temperature, soil, sunlight, and water all influence the makeup of herbs, as does the time of year they are harvested and the way they are handled after harvest. Therefore, different batches of herbs can vary unpredictably in strength.

Scientists need consistency to perform reproducible results in clinical trials. The lack of consistency in whole-herb products is one important reason that research and

And that wasn't the end of the story. After about 2 months of feeling better, when she came in to purchase another bottle, I suggested that she take the next step. With a smile, she told me that she had already taken it. "For the first time in my life I'm calm enough to practice yoga. I'm hoping that if I keep up the practice for 6 months or so, I'll have learned how to calm myself down. Then I won't need to take this herb."

Psychotherapy, yoga, tai chi, meditation, aerobic exercise, and biofeedback are some of the ways you might be able to gain a permanent sense of greater calm. And that calm will belong to you.

clinical testing of herbs lags behind that of conventional medications. It also is a reason that many pharmacists and physicians prefer drugs to whole herbs, as the dosage of drugs can be much more precisely controlled than the dosage or strength of herbs can be.

Traditional herbalists feel, smell, and taste herbs to determine their potency, but this practice would not go over well in the modern world. European herbal manufacturers invented a method that partially solves the problem of consistency: standardization of herbal extracts. In standardization, each batch of herbs is carefully processed to contain a certain fixed percentage of one or more ingredients that are used as "tags," or markers. Contrary to popular belief, these tags are not necessarily the active ingredients. They are simply "handles" to ensure batch-to-batch similarity.

In the case of kava, the kavalactones serve as the tags in the standardization process. Originally, standardized extracts of kava had a 70% concentration of kavalactones. More recently, a 30% concentration has become more popular.

The chemical constituents of herbs vary, depending on where and how the herb was grown; temperature, soil, sunlight, and water all influence the makeup of herbs.

The reason for this switch illustrates the limitations of standardized herbal extracts. Although kavalactones possess sedative properties, they apparently aren't the only active principles in kava. In clinical practice, 30% extracts seem to be more effective than 70% extracts when taken at a dose that provides the same amount of kavalactones. As we saw in chapter 1, this finding appears to indicate that other, unidentified active ingredients play a major role.

Because two batches of kava that are both standardized to the same percentage of kavalactones can vary in their content of these unknown ingredients, perfect consistency is not possible. This means that you can't be absolutely sure that two brands of kava are equally effective or even that one brand keeps a steady level of effectiveness from year to year. This is simply a problem with using herbs instead of drugs and one for which there is no ready solution.

The bottom line is that if one form of kava does not work for you, you might consider trying another, rather than giving up on the herb altogether. I also recommend buying a reputable brand. There is relatively little supervision over the content of herbal products, and many cases have been reported when the material inside the bottle was much weaker than the label indicated.

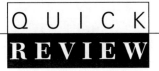

- Kava enjoys current popularity in Europe and the United States as a treatment for anxiety and is widely available in pharmacies; health-food, grocery, and mass merchandise stores; and by mail order.

- Make sure to buy a form of kava that is standardized to its kavalactone content. Usually, the product will be labeled to contain, for example, 30 to 70% kavalactones.

- To treat anxiety, the usual dose of kava should supply 20 to 70 mg of kavalactones 3 times daily. The total dose of kavalactones should not exceed 300 mg daily, and the course of treatment should not exceed 3 months. If anxiety persists, seek medical attention to rule out medical causes of anxiety, such as hyperthyroidism.

- Optimum results can take as long as 1 month to develop, so don't give up too soon. However, some people feel satisfactory relief quite quickly.

- Don't forget: Kava should not be regarded as a permanent solution. Once you feel more calm, find other ways to quiet your mind and heart, such as yoga, psychotherapy, tai chi, regular aerobic exercise, or meditation.

CHAPTER
SEVEN

Safety Issues

A s a pharmacist, I have a professional golden rule: Do no harm. Health-care professionals always try to find the best possible medicine with the fewest possible side effects for any given individual. We use what we call the risk-to-benefit ratio to evaluate various treatment options. In simple terms, we want the greatest benefit with the least amount of risk.

The same rule applies to herbal remedies. Although herbs are natural and often gentler, milder, and less toxic than drugs, they need to be treated with respect. Remember that any agent that has the ability to have a desirable effect, natural or synthetic, can also cause side effects at some higher dosage. In addition, some herbs cause side effects by themselves, whereas others might do so in combination with other medications or supplements.

This chapter examines kava's side effects, toxicity, and drug interactions as well as other special considerations you should be aware of before you decide whether to try kava.

Side Effects

Taken by itself in reasonable doses, kava is almost side-effect free. Several large, well-designed studies have found no serious side effects for kava and few mild ones. (However, one German journal reported four individual cases of unusual neurological side effects. See following discussion.)

Any food, drug, or herb can cause an allergic reaction in some people. Similarly, almost any herb can cause mild digestive distress. For this reason, these symptoms of mild gastrointestinal distress or mild allergic reactions are called *nonspecific* side effects. In general, the side effects reported for kava at reasonable doses have been nonspecific.

Although herbs are natural and often gentler, milder, and less toxic than drugs, they need to be treated with respect.

For example, one study of 4,049 individuals who took 105 mg daily of a 70% kavalactone extract for 7 weeks found side effects in 1.5% of cases. These were limited mainly to mild gastrointestinal complaints or allergic rashes. The symptoms stopped when the kavalactone extract was discontinued.[1] However, this study used a lower dose of kava than most people would actually use. In another study, 3,029 participants were given a more realistic dose of 800 mg daily of a 30% kavalactone extract for 4 weeks. This study yielded a 2.3% incidence of side effects, all of which again were mild (gastrointestinal discomfort, headache, dizziness, and allergic reactions).[2]

Interestingly, in a study of 100 people who received either placebo or 300 mg daily of a kava extract standardized to 70% kavalactones for 6 months, three times *more* side effects were reported in the placebo group than in the kava group.[3] It seems reasonable to assume that the side effects reported by the placebo group were actually symptoms of anxiety; and, if the placebo group's side effects were anxi-

ety symptoms, one might think that some of the side effects reported for kava might also be symptoms of anxiety.

Taken by itself in reasonable doses, kava is almost side-effect free.

Although headaches were noted in some of the participants taking 800 mg daily of 30% kava-lactones, this symptom is often reported in significant numbers by people given placebo and is not necessarily a true side effect.

Headaches have not been noted as a significant problem in any of the double-blind trials of kava.

One great advantage of kava, compared with conventional antianxiety medications, is that it doesn't seem to impair mental function. One clinical study tested coordination and reaction time in people taking either kava or placebo. In one study, participants were asked to keep a pointer at the midpoint between two shifting between parallel lines. In another, they were required to rapidly press a correct key in response to a signal. No statistically significant differences were found between the two groups' performance.

Although encouraging, this study does not prove that it is safe to drive a car or operate heavy machinery while taking kava. In fact, some authors, along with Germany's Commission E, advise caution in driving or operating other equipment while taking kava, just to be on the safe side. I'd recommend that you don't drive for a few hours after your first dose of kava. (See sidebar, Intoxicated on Kava). Some people are more sensitive to kava than others, and some people say that it makes them feel drowsy or even slightly intoxicated, especially during the first few days of using it. Once you've tried kava, you'll be better able to judge its effects on you.

The most notorious side effect of kava is a distinctive skin rash—so-called alligator skin—that can accompany heavy, long-term use. Fortunately, this side effect has not been reported for the moderate dosages we use for treating anxiety. *Kava dermopathy*, as the skin rash is called, was first reported by members of Captain James Cook's expedition in the South Pacific. Islanders who used kava excessively were seen to have dry, scaly eruptions, mainly on the palms, soles of the feet, forearms, shins, and back.

We don't have any reports of kava dermopathy (skin rash) occurring when kava is taken within the normal dosage range.

Because kava dermopathy resembles the rash of *pellagra* (a syndrome caused by niacin deficiency), it was first assumed that kava somehow interfered with the body's absorption of niacin. To test this theory, *niacinamide* (a form of niacin) was given to Tongans who had severe kava dermopathy in a double-blind placebo-controlled trial. Because the skin condition did not improve in those individuals receiving the niacinamide, researchers concluded that this dermopathy is not caused by niacin deficiency.[4]

It is still not clear why the eruption develops, but it disappears promptly when the kava is discontinued. Because no further research has taken place on this peculiar dermopathy, we don't know whether it indicates any other significant health risk. On a positive note, we don't have any reports of this dermopathy occurring when kava is taken within the normal dosage range.

Neurological Reactions:
A Rare Side Effect of Kava?

Four cases of bizarre neurological reactions to kava have been reported:[5]

1. A 28-year-old man had sharp spasms in the muscles of his neck and in his eyes that began about 90 minutes after taking 100 mg of kava extract. The spasms lasted about 40 minutes.
2. A 22-year-old woman experienced a similar reaction to the same product and was not taking any other medication.
3. A 63-year-old woman experienced a similar reaction after taking 150 mg of kava extract 3 times daily for 4 days.
4. A 76-year-old woman with early signs of Parkinson's disease reported a pronounced increase in the duration and number of episodes of impaired movement after switching from pharmaceuticals to 150 mg kava extract twice daily.

The last example suggests only that kava is not an effective treatment for Parkinson's disease. However, the others do raise concerns that kava might produce rare, unusual effects on the nervous system. It is also possible that the kava products these people took were contaminated with unknown ingredients. At present, it is not possible to make a definitive statement about these reactions, except that they are not common.

Toxicity

Side effects usually do not cause permanent harm, might or might not be related to the dose of the drug, and often occur in only some people who use them. *Toxicity* usually refers to a side effect that involves progressive damage to an organ or a part of the body, increases with the dose of the drug, and occurs in most people who use the drug.

Fortunately, kava seems to be relatively nontoxic. Tests involving rats and dogs showed no harmful effects when 70% kavalactone extract was given to them at doses of 20 mg/kg and 24 mg/kg daily. In humans, this would correspond to about 1,000 mg daily or more—a very high dose. Even at twice this dose in dogs and more than ten times this dose in rats, only mild signs of toxicity were observed.[6] However, extremely high doses of kava—700 mg/kg or more—were lethal in more than 50% of the mice tested.[7] In humans, this would work out to more than 100 times the maximum recommended daily dose of kava. The safety margin of kava appears to be very great.

It is probably safe to say that even at several times the recommended dose of kava, immediately obvious harmful effects do not occur.

Another factor to consider is that kava has been used traditionally for hundreds of years in fairly high doses. Large quantities of kava beverage—the equivalent of several grams of kavalactones—are commonly consumed in kava's traditional context. Thus, it is probably safe to say that even at several times the recommended dose of kava, immediately obvious harmful effects do not occur.

Long-Term Safety

As with most herbs and drugs, the long-term safety of kava has not been evaluated. One study did find signs of possible toxicity with a very high dosage of kava. This study

Intoxicated on Kava

A motorist was arrested in Utah for driving erratically. Police thought he was drunk, because he staggered, answered questions slowly, and his speech was slurred. When a breath test found no evidence of alcohol, they were confused. Ultimately, they discovered that he was under the influence of 16 cups of kava. Even though kava is legal, he was convicted for driving while intoxicated, the first such case in the United States.[8]

We know from experiences in the South Pacific that when used to excess, kava is definitely intoxicating. Keep this in mind when using kava for anxiety. At proper doses it should be safe, but I definitely recommend discovering how you react before getting behind the wheel.

followed Australian aboriginals who habitually consumed more than 100 times the normal dose of kava, a dosage that, according to the animal studies just described, falls within the toxic zone. These people experienced many detrimental physiological changes as noted by laboratory tests (to be specific, decreased blood levels of albumin, plasma protein, urea, and bilirubin, accompanied by hematuria, decreased platelet count, and enlarged red blood cells).[9] However, because this population also consumed large doses of alcohol and smoked cigarettes, we don't know whether their poor health was due to the kava or the preexisting alcohol and cigarette abuse. Also, it is hard to say how this study relates, if at all, to anyone consuming kava in reasonable amounts for shorter periods of time.

To be on the safe side, as well as to avoid psychological dependence, Germany's Commission E recommends limiting kava treatment to no longer than 3 months at a time.

Addiction

Traditionally, kava has been used not only for spiritual or ceremonial reasons but also recreationally in the way that other societies have used alcohol. This history gives rise to concerns that kava might be abused as a "party herb" in modern Western culture. The evidence on kava and addiction is mixed. One study appeared to show some potential for kava addiction in mice.[10] On the other hand, kava has been used clinically in Europe for a number of years without any evidence of addiction surfacing.

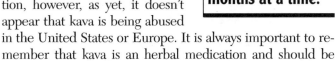

To be on the safe side, Germany's Commission E recommends limiting kava treatment to no longer than 3 months at a time.

We know that extremely high doses of kava can cause inebriation, however, as yet, it doesn't appear that kava is being abused in the United States or Europe. It is always important to remember that kava is an herbal medication and should be treated with respect.

Drug Interactions

A fair amount of evidence suggests that it's not a good idea to combine kava with benzodiazepines or other antianxiety medications. At least one case of severe mental disorientation, apparently resulting from combining Xanax (a benzodiazepine) with kava extract, has been reported.[11] This was a 54-year-old man who had been taking Xanax as well as the ulcer drug cimetidine and the prostate drug terazocin. He then started to take kava, and after 3 days he wound up in the hospital in a semi-coma.

It is quite possible that the other drugs he was taking played a role in his condition. However, because research

Beth and Ann's Story

For any treatment—pharmaceutical or herbal—side effects are unpredictable because each person is so different that similar treatments can produce vastly different results. The story of Beth and Ann, 20- and 22-year-old sisters, is a good case in point. Both came into the pharmacy one day with an article from a popular magazine that extolled the virtues of kava, and they wanted to buy some to help them with the high pressure of college. "It's all natural—what have we got to lose?" I heard Ann ask Beth as they purchased the kava.

I didn't see them again until spring break from school, when Beth came into the pharmacy with a prescription for Fiorinal for her headaches. As I was giving her a consultation on her new prescription, I inquired as to any medicines, vitamins, or herbs she might be taking. "A daily vitamin and kava for stress," was Beth's reply. I asked her what she thought might be the cause of her headaches, to which she replied,

leads us to think that kava affects the same nervous system mechanisms that are also affected by benzodiazepines, barbiturates, and other antianxiety medications, it seems reasonable that combined treatment could cause exaggerated and extreme effects. For this reason, Germany's Commission E advises caution when combining kava with any central nervous system depressant.

Warning: Benzodiazepines and other antianxiety medications remain in the body for some time after you've ceased taking them. Interactions can occur as long as the drug remains in your body. For this reason, as well as be-

"Too much stress, I guess. Now I'm on both kava and this new Fiorinal prescription."

Questioning a bit further, I found out that both Ann and Beth had been taking kava for their college anxieties. Ann was having no problems, but Beth had developed headaches ever since she started the kava. She hadn't made the connection, but I did. I asked Beth whether she would be willing to stop taking the kava for a few days to see whether her headaches would subside on their own before starting her prescription medication. "But kava's all natural. How could it give me headaches?" she asked. However, because I was persistent, she reluctantly agreed. A few days later, she reported back to me that it had worked. The headaches were gone.

The moral of the story is that even natural remedies can cause side effects in some people. Everyone is unique. Although they were members of the same family, Beth experienced headaches and Ann didn't. It pays to pay attention.

cause of the possibility of dangerous withdrawal symptoms, never switch from a benzodiazepine or other psychoactive medication to kava without a physician's supervision.

Because alcohol is also a depressant, the same caution applies to combining kava and alcohol. One study showed that high doses of alcohol enhanced the toxicity of moderate doses of kava in mice.[12]

Interestingly, one study in humans suggests that kava might actually counter some of the performance-related deficits caused by alcohol consumption. However, this is not to say that it's a good idea to combine kava and alcohol; you should not combine kava with any sedative drug (including alcohol). Because we don't have all the answers, it is best to err on the side of caution.

Never switch from a benzodiazepine or other psychoactive medication to kava without a physician's supervision.

We also don't know whether it's really safe to combine kava with other psychoactive herbs, such as valerian or St. John's wort. No studies on these inter-herb interactions have been done. Although many herbalists recommend these combinations without any reported problems, some authors recommend avoiding these combinations until complete safety studies are available. This doesn't mean that it is definitely bad to take these herbs together but rather that we don't yet have safety studies on these combinations.

Is Kava Safe During Pregnancy and While Nursing?

For any drug or herb, ethical and liability concerns make it difficult to do the kind of studies that would establish safety for pregnant and nursing women. Because of this lack of research, we usually don't know whether drugs or medications are safe for either pregnant or nursing women. This is certainly the case with kava. Although no clinical evidence suggests that kava causes any particular harm during pregnancy and nursing, Germany's Commission E monograph warns against its use under those circumstances as a matter of prudence. As previously mentioned, with any herb or medication, it is always best to err on the side of safety.

Is Kava Safe for Children?

Whether the use of kava is safe for children is yet another question that cannot be answered with certainty because all the studies of kava have been performed with adults.

We know that historically kava has been given to children to treat whooping cough, but no historical reports have indicated the safety of, or any side effects from, this treatment. As is true with other herbs used for children, reports and safety indications are still largely absent.

Is Kava Safe for Those with Liver or Kidney Disease?

Drugs are processed through the liver and kidneys. In people with severe impairment of the liver or kidneys, drugs might not be processed normally and might build up to unusually high and thus dangerous levels. We don't know whether this would happen with kava, but until we find out, I wouldn't recommend kava for people with severe liver or kidney disease except under a physician's supervision.

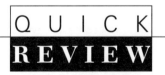

QUICK
REVIEW

- The side-effect and safety profile of kava is quite good. It occasionally causes mild side effects such as stomach upset, but no serious side effects have been reported for ordinary dosages. However, long-term use of high doses of kava (400 mg or more of kavalactones daily over a period of months or years) can cause a peculiar scaly rash. This rash goes away when you stop taking kava.

- Excessive use of kava can cause intoxication. Even when using it properly, I would advise against getting behind the wheel of a car until you are sure how it affects you.

- Kava should not be combined with alcohol, benzodiazepines, or other sedatives.

- The safety of kava for young children, pregnant or nursing women, and those with severe liver and kidney disease has not been established. In such cases, it's best to err on the side of caution.

How Kava Compares with Conventional Medications

I n chapter 5, we discussed the evidence that kava is an effective treatment for anxiety. This safe herb begins to work in about 1 to 8 weeks and appears to provide significant benefits with few side effects. European physicians often try it first for those with anxiety.

However, most U.S. physicians use drugs in the benzodiazepine family to treat anxiety. If you are considering trying kava instead, you will naturally want to know how it compares to this standard approach. In this chapter, we will examine the results of scientific studies that have compared kava against conventional drugs. This is a short chapter because, as yet, few studies have been conducted. No doubt, in future editions of this book, this chapter will have expanded to cover the intensive research that is under way at the present time.

Effectiveness Comparisons

To date, only one significant double-blind study has looked at the relative effectiveness of kava extract and conventional pharmaceuticals. This was the Woelk study, a 6-week double-blind trial enrolling 174 individuals with anxiety.[1] The results showed no difference in effectiveness between the treatments.

The individuals selected for this trial had average HAM-A scores of about 28. As you might remember from

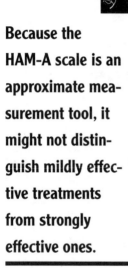

chapter 5, the HAM-A scale rates the level of anxiety, with higher numbers indicating more severe symptoms. A HAM-A score of 28 represents a moderate level of anxiety.

Because the HAM-A scale is an approximate measurement tool, it might not distinguish mildly effective treatments from strongly effective ones.

Participants accepted into the trial received either 100 mg of a standard kava extract 3 times daily, 5 mg of oxazepam 3 times daily, or 3 mg of bromazepam 3 times daily. Oxazepam is a benzodiazepine drug that is no longer widely used for anxiety. Bromazepam is another benzodiazepine drug that is not available in the United States but is widely used for anxiety in some parts of Europe.

Over the 6 weeks of the trial, all three treatments produced approximately an equal amount of benefits. The average HAM-A scores fell by about 45% in all three groups, and from a rigorous mathematical point of view, there was no difference in the outcomes.

Besides this trial, at least two double-blind studies have compared synthetic kavain, one of the active ingredients of kava, against standard benzodiazepine drugs.[2,3] However, because their results don't directly apply to whole kava extract that you can buy in pharmacies and health-food stores, I don't describe their results here.

Is Kava Really As Effective As Benzodiazepines?

The Woelk study was large enough for its results to be statistically meaningful, and it was conducted according to reasonably good scientific standards. However, its results are a bit surprising. It appears to suggest that kava is just as effective as benzodiazepine treatment. This is not what one would really expect. Most doctors who use kava feel that it is somewhat less effective than benzodiazepines (see chapter 5 and the following discussion). What is the explanation for this discrepancy?

A close look at this study will identify several possibilities. First, the dose of oxazepam used was two to four times lower than what is usually recommended for moderate anxiety. The comparison wasn't really fair. A proper dose of oxazepam might have worked much better.

Fortunately, the amount of bromazepam used was in the realm of standard practice. If kava is truly just as effective as this medication, it should be a strong advertisement for the herb. However, there is another, more fundamental reason that kava might have seemed just as powerful as benzodiazepines in this study even though it probably isn't: the coarseness of the HAM-A rating scale. What do I mean by this?

When medical researchers study the effects of drugs and herbs that lower cholesterol, for example, they are able to measure cholesterol levels very precisely. Even the smallest difference shows up on the laboratory machine that reports the amount of cholesterol in the blood.

By comparison, the HAM-A scale is a crude measurement tool. It relies on very rough estimates of anxiety symptoms on a 0 to 4 scale. This kind of rough estimate might not be able to pick out the difference between a mildly effective treatment and a strongly effective one.

Here's an analogy: Suppose you own a very cheap stopwatch that displays time only in 30-second intervals. Your stopwatch should be perfectly good enough to show a difference in speed between an automobile and a snail. However, it wouldn't be of much use comparing the running times of athletes. The difference between a good high-school athlete and a world-champion sprinter would probably be less than 30 seconds, so, as far as your cheap watch was concerned, one time would be just as good as the other.

The consensus appears to be that kava is a milder treatment than standard drugs, but for many people that very mildness might be perfect.

Similarly, the HAM-A scale can detect differences between kava (or benzodiazepines) and placebo treatment because the difference in effectiveness is very large. However, it might not be able to distinguish between a treatment that works pretty well and another that works very well. If kava makes people feel "somewhat less anxious" and benzodiazepine drugs make them feel "definitely less anxious," the HAM-A rating scale might not be able to tell the difference.

For this reason, even if kava and full doses of benzodiazepine drugs were found to produce equivalent changes in HAM-A scores, it would certainly be possible that they really weren't equally effective. Actually, few participants who have tried both treatments, or doctors who prescribe them would claim that they are equally powerful. The consensus appears to be that kava is a milder treatment than standard drugs, but for many people that very mildness might be perfect. Do you really need your anxiety taken away altogether, or would an herb that "takes the edge off" be just as good (or even better)? That is for you to decide.

What Doctors Say

Typically, doctors who prescribe kava feel that it is not as effective as benzodiazepine drugs. One family physician who was interviewed for this book expressed it as follows: "I basically use benzodiazepines and kava for two different kinds of people. For folks having a difficult time coping with some rough spots in their lives, I find that benzodiazepines may be overkill. I like to recommend the gentler approach of kava. I've tried kava myself, so I have a sense of how it works. But for people with severe anxiety, a benzodiazepine drug may be necessary, at least until therapy or other treatments have a chance to work."

Steven Bratman, M.D., also feels that kava is a good option for people with mild to moderate anxiety. He says, "It often appears to be very helpful for people with a constant low level of anxiety, anxiety that's irritating but not disabling. People tell me that the surface of the sea is smoothed out, so to speak.

"I remember a student from a farming town who was finding the experience of life in an urban university rather jangling. He couldn't sleep well, and he felt nervous most of the day.

"He had started to drink wine, but I suggested he try kava instead. It worked well for him. I'm a lot happier having him rely on kava rather than alcohol, although I'd rather he find a way to get by without having to take anything at all.

"However, kava does not seem to work when (to use the same metaphor) there's a storm on the sea. I have seen at least 20 individuals with severe anxiety who came

Kava Versus Standard Drugs:
One Psychiatrist's Opinion

When asked his views on kava and standard drugs in the treatment of anxiety, one psychiatrist commented, "I'm a specialist, so I naturally see more intense cases than your average doctor. When individuals have massive, severe anxiety, family practitioners are likely to send them to me. I know for a fact that kava is not strong enough to help them because many of them have tried it already, and it didn't work. When I give them high doses of benzodiazepines, it's like another world. Those drugs have problems, but they really work.

to me after kava failed. The herb just didn't touch it, while benzodiazepines worked like magic.

"I suspect that kava may be about as strong as BuSpar (buspirone). This drug also works gradually and doesn't handle severe anxiety. I'd like to see some studies performed that compare these two treatments, but I usually offer one or the other when people come to me with mild to moderate anxiety. When people are anxious enough to need benzodiazepines, I usually refer them to a specialist."

Side-Effect Comparisons

One of the main reasons that people try herbs is because herbs frequently cause fewer side effects than drugs used for the same purpose. For example, unlike Prozac, St. John's wort does not cause sexual problems, headache, or sleeplessness. However, in the case of anxiety, the standard options don't cause many side effects, either. Because benzodiazepine drugs cause relatively few unpleas-

"But the truth is that most people who complain that they feel anxious aren't as bad off as those people with severe anxiety. People with more mild to moderate anxiety often tell me that kava helps them a lot. And I'm all for whatever works. I recommend exercise, meditation, and psychotherapy, too. None of those will be successful for overwhelming anxiety, but that's not most people's problem. What I say is this: Kava for the smaller anxieties, benzodiazepines for the bigger anxieties. It makes sense to me. If you give Xanax to someone with mild anxiety, it's overkill."

ant symptoms, kava might not have a particular advantage in this regard.

In the Woelk study, few side effects were reported in any group. Four people taking bromazepam reported fatigue; a few people taking oxazepam experienced fatigue, headache, or vertigo; and one individual given kava spoke of mild digestive distress and another reported decreased motivation. Overall, the physicians felt that side effects were minimal in all three groups. Keeping in mind that the oxazepam dose in this study was unrealistically low, it appears that kava and benzodiazepines might have a similarly insignificant side-effect profile.

However, kava might have an edge over benzodiazepines in one regard. When taken in high doses, these medications can impair reaction time and mental function. Preliminary evidence suggests that kava does not present this problem.

In a double-blind placebo-controlled study, 12 subjects were tested regarding their memory, reaction time, and

Ben's Story

Ben had been getting his prescription for Valium refilled off and on for the past 6 months. He had a high-pressure management position within a computer technology firm and suffered from a lot of work-related stress and anxiety. He came to me to request another refill, but with the following comments: "I'm not sure I should have this Valium refilled again. It does take the edge off my anxiety, but I've found that I'm not as mentally sharp when I take it. My math and my computer skills go downhill, and it's getting me into trouble at work. It's a vicious cycle—I'm anxious about work, so I take Valium, which makes me perform badly, which, makes me anxious about work.

"I haven't taken any Valium for 2 weeks. But I still haven't dug out from under the pile of work on my desk. I'm feeling so anxious I'd really like to get some Valium, but that will just dig me deeper in. I need a different solution."

Ben was not a regular user of Valium and had been off the medication long enough to be sure that it was out of his system. Thus, I felt it was safe to recommend that he try kava in-

attention span while taking 75 mg of oxazepam daily (about twice the usual dose), 600 mg of standardized kava extract daily (also about twice the usual dose), or placebo.[4,5]

The results were striking. According to a variety of standard psychological tests, oxazepam was found to significantly impair mental functioning and reaction time compared to placebo. However, while taking kava, participants scored at least as well on the tests as when they were given placebo.

stead of Valium for the next several weeks. If it didn't work, I suggested that he check back with his physician.

I didn't hear back from him again, until he came into the store several months later to buy some toothpaste. He saw me behind the counter and came up specially to give me a report. "That kava you recommended sure does work for me," he said. "It keeps me calm without dulling my brain."

However, he hadn't become a permanent user of kava. "After I cleared out my in-box, I got back into the swing of things and quit taking it. I feel like I'm back to my old self again and out of trouble at work! I don't want to be dependent on anything."

I suggested that he take a stress-reduction class to help prepare him to deal with stressful times in the future, and he agreed to start.

Did kava really impair his mind to a lesser extent, or was Ben's experience just due to the power of suggestion? Without good, solid evidence, we really don't know.

Actually, on a couple of measures, kava seemed to increase mental function slightly. However, the change was so small that it could have been due to chance, and the researchers described it as insignificant. Nonetheless, this study has been widely misreported as proving that kava actually improved mental function. That is stretching the results too far. (Another mistake is that two separate published reports of the same study are widely referenced as two distinct studies that confirm each other!)

Furthermore, the dose of the benzodiazepine drug used was considerably higher than normal. At the present time, it is not clear that benzodiazepine drugs, when taken appropriately, impair mental function more than kava.

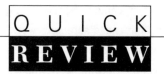

- One study suggests that kava might be as effective as standard benzodiazepine drugs. However, most physicians feel that compared to standard benzodiazepine drugs, kava is a gentler treatment that takes the edge off anxiety rather than making it go away entirely.
- Neither kava nor benzodiazepine drugs cause many side effects. However, there is some evidence that benzodiazepines can impair mental function and reaction time while kava does not.

Other Alternative
Treatments
for Anxiety

I f you are one of the estimated 50 million adults
in the United States alone who suffer from anxiety, you might have already tried a variety of self-
treatments, therapies, and medications to get relief. I
noted earlier that the benzodiazepine antianxiety medications make up 5% of all prescriptions in the United
States today. Kava, we learned, is an effective and safe
herbal treatment for anxiety that is not severe. This
chapter addresses other alternative therapies for anxiety,
including valerian. It also discusses in more detail the
benefits of psychotherapy, either alone or in combination
with other treatments. Anxiety is often a condition with
many causes that can benefit from a variety of treatments. The therapies discussed in this chapter are tools
that can be useful, either alone or in combination with
medication or kava.

Valerian

The herb valerian is more fully discussed in chapter 10 as a treatment for insomnia. However, because it is also used for anxiety, I will briefly discuss it here.

Anxiety is often a condition with many causes that can benefit from a variety of treatments.

Valerian (*Valeriana officinalis*) is a tall perennial herb with a sharp, distinctive odor loved by cats. (See figure 3). The roots of the valerian plant are used for medicinal purposes, most often as a sedative and sleep aid. As far back as the second century A.D., the Greek physician Galen recommended valerian for insomnia, and it's been a popular sedative in Europe since the sixteenth century.

Our understanding of how valerian works is incomplete. Some evidence suggests that valerian affects levels of gamma-amino-butyric acid (GABA) in the brain. GABA, as you might recall from chapter 4, is a naturally occurring amino acid that appears to be related to anxiety levels. Conventional antianxiety medications in the benzodiazepine family, such as Valium, are known to affect GABA receptors in the brain, and valerian might work similarly. Studies suggest that it either stimulates GABA receptors[1,2] or increases GABA concentrations.[3] However, these findings have been disputed.[4] More studies are needed to complete our understanding of how valerian works.

Until 1950, valerian was officially listed in the U.S. National Formulary as a sleep aid and antianxiety agent. German health authorities officially recognize it today as useful for "nervous tension; difficulty in getting to sleep; and nervous, cramp-like pains in the gastrointestinal re-

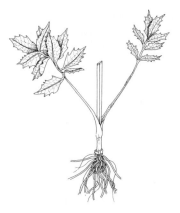

Figure 3. *Valerian*

gion." Thus, although valerian is probably more useful for insomnia (see chapter 10), it is sometimes recommended as a treatment for anxiety as well.

Unfortunately, the scientific research for valerian's use in anxiety is almost nonexistent. Most of the research on valerian pertains to its use in insomnia. However, one study has indicated that valerian can reduce feelings of anxiety. This double-blind study of 48 subjects exposed normal, healthy individuals to intense short-term stress and measured their physiological responses. Each of these individuals received one of the following: placebo, a beta-blocker (a class of drugs that slows heart rate), valerian, or a combination of valerian and beta-blocker. Valerian reduced subjective feelings of anxiety but not pulse rate. Subjects receiving the beta-blocker (alone or with valerian) showed decreased pulse rates as well, as one might expect, as that is the major effect of beta-blockers.[5] This suggests that valerian might be useful for short-term stresses such as performance anxiety (stage fright). However, more research is needed to help us understand how useful valerian is for anxiety.

A typical dose of valerian is 2 to 3 g twice daily, usually taken in capsule form to hide the odor as much as possible.

Valerian appears to be safe when taken at normal doses, and the U.S. Food and Drug Administration lists it on its GRAS (generally recognized as safe) list. Except for the unpleasant odor, valerian causes no serious side effects in most people. However, some individuals experience mild gastrointestinal distress, and there have been rare reports of individuals developing a mild stimulant effect from valerian—the exact opposite of what it's expected to do.

The roots of the valerian plant are used for medicinal purposes, most often as a sedative and sleep aid.

Valerian does not appear to impair driving ability or produce morning drowsiness when taken at night.[6] However, it might impair attention for a couple of hours after it is taken. Thus, it isn't a good idea to drive immediately afterward. As with most herbs and many drugs, its safety has not been established for young children, pregnant and nursing women, and those with severe liver or kidney disease.

In practice, valerian's effects on anxiety are mild at best. Valerian is definitely not as strong as prescription antianxiety medications and is probably not as strong as kava.

Warning: Never attempt to switch from a medication for anxiety to an herbal alternative except under a physician's supervision. Taking herbs or medications are only two of many possible ways to treat anxiety. Although both herbs and prescription drugs can be extremely helpful, there are many other things you can do to reduce stress in your life and improve your own health and coping skills. The rest of this chapter will give you some ideas for other treatments.

Alternative Therapies

More than one in three Americans use some form of alternative treatment for health problems. Anxiety is the second most common reason for using alternative treatments (the first is chronic pain). In addition to herbs, anxiety sufferers frequently seek relief through the alternative therapies of massage, acupuncture, relaxation techniques, yoga, and meditation.

It's easy to get lost in the world of alternative therapies. Which ones work, and which ones don't? A good way to get started is to ask your therapist or physician for recommendations.

Massage, acupuncture, relaxation techniques, yoga, and meditation are readily available in most cities and regions and can provide stress relief for the body and mind. Unlike kava, all of these treatments can be combined quite safely with any medications you are taking. In fact, it might be that combining these techniques with your prescription or herbal medications will improve your results and help you minimize your dosage.

There are no studies or good scientific evidence that these treatments are effective

Massage, acupuncture, relaxation techniques, yoga, and meditation are readily available in most cities and can provide stress relief for the body and mind.

for anxiety disorders. However, many people swear by each of these methods. You only need to receive a good massage to know that anything that helps your body relax can help your mind relax, too.

Washing Away the Stress

A retired surgeon friend of mine related to me the healthful wonders of his newfound pastimes of yoga, meditation, and massage. "Why didn't I do this 20 years ago? These techniques that I looked down upon all these years bring so much to my life now. They remove the tension and relax and revitalize me. I wish I had started these practices during my working years. It would have helped me cope with the load of anxiety I experienced from the tremendous pressures of medicine. Now, a week doesn't go by that I don't participate in two or more of these life-giving practices. I feel so at ease now. I recommend them to all my friends. . . . I'm hooked."

Lifestyle Changes

Lifestyle changes are sometimes the last thing we want when we're already feeling anxious. Change makes most of us tense, and some of us find it especially difficult to change our lifestyles. However, a balanced, healthful style of living can do a great deal to relieve anxiety permanently. As difficult as change is, it can be worth it.

You don't have to wait for your health-care provider to ask you the following questions; you can do your own self-assessment right now. So here we go. I'll play the physician, psychotherapist, or alternative health-care provider and ask, "Do you exercise? Do you eat a healthful diet? Do you drink alcohol, and if so, how much? Do you drink coffee, and if so, how much? What's your stress level at work? How's your social life? How's your home life?"

We learned in chapter 3 that too much caffeine can cause anxiety and that too much alcohol and a poor diet can stress the body and mind. Besides a good diet, coping-

Cindy's Story

Recently, I helped teach a class in stress management. The purpose of the class was to help participants cut down on their antianxiety medication. When we gave people in the class a list of life's stressors, one attendee named Cindy was amazed. After adding up the stressors in her life, she realized that her lifestyle would make anyone anxious. "I have to make some real changes if I want to get off Valium."

Cindy realized that she was overcommitted. Besides taking care of her aging mother and her two children, she had a full-time job, volunteered at a homeless shelter, held a position on a city planning advisory committee, and led a Cub Scout den. It was simply too much. "I have to realize my limits and say 'no' sometimes."

It's important to look at your life and see what you can change to reduce your stress level. Don't count on a drug or an herb to make an impossible lifestyle manageable. Sometimes you simply have to find real-life solutions to real-life problems.

and stress-management skills are equally important. Including time for exercise, meditation, or relaxation in your daily routine can help you handle the unavoidable stresses in your day.

Psychotherapy

Psychotherapy can be an important tool in the treatment of all forms of anxiety, including general anxiety disorder, situational anxiety, panic attacks, phobias, obsessive-compulsive behavior, and post-traumatic stress disorder. If you think you have one of these more severe anxiety conditions (as explained further in chapter 2), your physician or therapist can best guide you.

In generalized anxiety disorders, psychotherapy can help uncover underlying psychological causes. We can be suffering from stubborn emotional complexes that simply cannot be alleviated by taking a medication. A skilled psychotherapist can help unravel these psychological binds that keep us from living life fully. Anxiety can be thought of as a "tightness in the mind" and, often, in the body as well. As we loosen ourselves from our emotional bondage, the feelings of anxiety can lessen.

A skilled psychotherapist can help unravel these psychological binds that keep us from living life fully.

Psychotherapy can provide us with coping skills for life. The benefits of therapy can extend far beyond the immediate situation or cause of the anxiety, and that is a blessing. However, psychotherapy is a process, and it requires commitment and time. For these reasons, it is often combined with medications that can provide more immediate relief while the underlying problems are being resolved.

Other Supplements

As a pharmacist, I have some final comments for you regarding other often-asked-about herbal and nutritional supplements for anxiety. Those that I mention here have no real scientific evidence as to their effectiveness, but they are widely used, and some people report that they help.

Besides kava and valerian, herbs that are frequently used for anxiety include lemon balm, hops, skullcap, and lady's slipper. Lemon balm is a pleasant-smelling herb (unlike valerian) that is generally available in tincture and tea forms. I personally prefer the tea form because the aroma and taste are soothing in themselves. Lemon balm is said to relieve spasms in the digestive tract and gently promote sleep. It is often combined with valerian, hops, or both to ease tension, help digestion, and treat insomnia.

As we loosen ourselves from our emotional bondage, our feelings of anxiety can lessen.

Medicinal hops are the same hops used in the preparation of beer to enhance its flavor. Workers in hops fields tend to become relaxed and tired more rapidly than can be explained by the direct physical work, and although dried hops are not as powerful, they do seem to possess some of the same effects. High-hopped beers like India pale ale are known for their sedative effects, independent of their alcohol content. Despite the lack of scientific evidence for effectiveness, lemon balm and hops are approved by Germany's Commission E to help nervousness and related conditions and should be taken according to label instructions. Both are believed to be essentially nontoxic when used at recommended doses.

Skullcap is another herb that has been used historically to relieve anxiety. It is often used today to help relieve the nervous tension and irritability of premenstrual syndrome (PMS). It is most often available as a tincture or in combination with other herbs in a product formulation. However, little safety information is available on skullcap. Overdosage reportedly can cause mental confusion and other neurological symptoms, and there are concerns over possible liver toxicity that are yet to be proven.

Even less information is available on the herb lady's slipper. It is often used for anxiety and insomnia, but its safety is not established.

Some alternative practitioners suggest simply taking GABA as an amino acid–supplement for anxiety. The rationale behind this is that GABA is known to play a central role in anxiety. However, there is no scientific evidence that orally ingested GABA gets to any place in the body where it can do any good. Finally, a few unimpressive studies have reported that supplementation with selenium (200 mcg daily), flaxseed oil (2 to 6 tablespoon daily), and a general multivitamin can help relieve anxiety symptoms in some people.

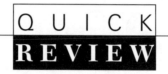

QUICK REVIEW

- Valerian is another safe herbal alternative that is also suggested as a treatment for anxiety taken at a dosage of 2 to 3 g twice daily. However, there is little scientific evidence on its effectiveness for anxiety. It is more commonly used for insomnia.

- Lifestyle changes can help improve the external factors that can fuel anxiety and add to our overall health. Psychotherapy is an important therapeutic tool for those whose anxiety has a basis in emotional conflicts. These tools require commitment and time but can give lasting, wide-ranging benefits. They can also be an important addition to any medications or herbs you are taking.

- Other herbs sometimes recommended for anxiety include lemon balm, hops, skullcap, and lady's slipper. However, there is next to no evidence that they are effective.

- Whereas lemon balm and hops are believed to be safe when used in reasonable doses, the safety of skullcap and lady's slipper has not been established.

- Other supplements, such as GABA, selenium, flaxseed oil, and multivitamins, have been suggested as aids for treating anxiety, but there is no scientific evidence at this time on the effectiveness of these remedies.

Insomnia

As we saw in chapter 2, anxious people frequently suffer from insomnia or other forms of disturbed sleep. Actually, it's a vicious cycle. Anxiety can disturb a person's sleep, and the fatigue resulting from not sleeping can also create feelings of anxiety. Some kind of treatment might be necessary to break the cycle and restore both sleep and calm.

Besides standard medications used for sleep, several natural sleep aids can be helpful for insomnia. Valerian (mentioned in chapter 9 as an alternative treatment for anxiety) is the most well-known herb for insomnia. Melatonin, a hormone that's available over the counter, is also a popular sleeping aid, especially for those suffering from jet lag. Finally, as we saw in chapter 5, kava is sometimes used for the same purpose.

This chapter briefly discusses conventional as well as herbal treatments for insomnia.

What Is Insomnia?

Need we define insomnia? Most of us have probably experienced insomnia at least once in our lives, and if you've spent even one night listening to the clock ticking relentlessly away while sleep eluded you, you're not likely to forget the feeling. Insomnia is a very common problem. More than one-third of adults in the United States alone suffer from it. It is not only annoying, but by depriving us of the sleep that we need for our health and general well-being, insomnia can seriously impair our everyday functioning and even our lives. Lack of sleep is a major factor contributing to automobile accidents as well as crises such as the Three Mile Island nuclear accident and the Exxon *Valdez* oil spill.[1]

Insomnia is a term that describes a variety of sleep disruptions and disturbances. The main kinds of insomnia are the following:[2]

- Difficulty falling asleep
- Difficulty staying asleep
- Waking up early in the morning and not being able to fall back to sleep
- Waking up after a full night of sleep but not feeling rested

If you recognize yourself in any of these descriptions of insomnia, you might have already found out that your mental, emotional, and physical health can suffer because of it. If insomnia is an ongoing problem in your life, you should be aware that your well-being and health are compromised from sleep deficits in three ways:

- Impaired mental abilities
- Disturbed moods
- Altered immune functions

It's shocking to some of us to realize the extent to which the seemingly minor annoyance of insomnia can affect our lives. The first aftereffect from insomnia, impaired mental abilities, has wide-ranging consequences. Fatigue-induced impairment of judgment is a factor in many accidents on the highways and at work.[3] Mental function is typically the

Insomnia is a very common problem. More than one-third of adults in the United States alone suffer from it.

first thing to decline when the body is deprived of sleep. The second aftereffect, disturbed moods, can take the form of irritability, mild depression, or anxiety. Finally, if sleep loss persists, eventually the third aftereffect, altered immune functions, can result. At this point, your body's immune functions suffer, making you more vulnerable to illnesses. It's really true that you need your 8 hours of sleep, but too many people go without.

The Normal Sleep Cycle

To understand the mental and cognitive symptoms of insomnia, it is useful first to know the phases of the normal sleep cycle. As we sleep, we go through a progression of phases. The two major phases of sleep are called rapid-eye-movement (REM) and non-rapid-eye-movement (NREM) sleep. Phases of sleep can be captured as particular brain wave patterns on a test called an electroencephalogram (or EEG).

When you are awake, an EEG typically reveals a pattern dominated by beta brain waves, which are very fast waves that signal alertness. As you fall asleep, your brain waves slow down, and other waves begin to dominate, including alpha 1, theta, and finally the very slow delta waves. Your heart rate slows as well.

The most restful and restorative phase of sleep is reached when the body and brain enter the deep, slow-wave, NREM stage, usually within 90 minutes of falling asleep. About one-fifth of normal sleep is spent in this most restful phase.

REM, the other phase of sleep, is often called *paradoxical sleep.* During this phase, which we enter for several brief periods during the night, our bodies are active. Our heart rate increases, our muscles twitch, and our eyelids flicker. If you've ever watched a cat or dog twitch in its sleep, you've seen what REM sleep looks like. This is the phase during which we dream. Each night, we spend a total of about 90 minutes in REM sleep. REM sleep appears to be extremely important, for when individuals are intentionally deprived of it in laboratory experiments, many symptoms develop, from grogginess to outright hallucinations. NREM sleep is also essential to help rest and restore us.

The most restful and restorative phase of sleep is reached when the body and brain enter the deep, slow-wave, NREM stage.

What Causes Insomnia?

Possible causes of insomnia include various mental and physical states, specific foods and medicines, lifestyle and environmental factors, and hormonal fluctuations. Anxiety itself can make a good night's sleep difficult because anxious people can have trouble falling asleep, and, once asleep, they might wake up many times throughout the night. The following pages discuss some factors that can interfere with your sleeping patterns.

Psychological, Age, and Hormonal Factors

The most common causes of insomnia are psychological influences—anxiety, tension, and depression. The hormonal changes that come with pregnancy, menopause, and age can also cause restless nights. (For many reasons, people tend to sleep less deeply as they get older.)

These factors can easily interact with one another. For example, hormonal fluctuations can lead to mood swings, and aging can be accompanied by life changes that are stressful in themselves.

Medications

Sometimes medications can cause sleep disturbance as an unwanted side effect. Some common drugs known to cause insomnia include oral contraceptives, too

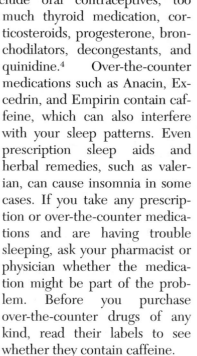

If you take any prescription or over-the-counter medications and are having trouble sleeping, ask your pharmacist or physician whether the medication might be part of the problem.

much thyroid medication, corticosteroids, progesterone, bronchodilators, decongestants, and quinidine.[4] Over-the-counter medications such as Anacin, Excedrin, and Empirin contain caffeine, which can also interfere with your sleep patterns. Even prescription sleep aids and herbal remedies, such as valerian, can cause insomnia in some cases. If you take any prescription or over-the-counter medications and are having trouble sleeping, ask your pharmacist or physician whether the medication might be part of the problem. Before you purchase over-the-counter drugs of any kind, read their labels to see whether they contain caffeine.

Diet, Alcohol, and Caffeine

Foods that are hard to digest can contribute to insomnia, especially if they're eaten close to bedtime. Some people find that their sleep is disturbed by eating spicy or high-fat foods within a couple of hours of going to bed.

The most notorious "foods" that disrupt sleep are alcohol and caffeine, both of which alter the body's sleep cycle. Many people use alcohol as a sleep aid, but its use—especially for persistent insomnia caused by an underlying psychological or physical problem—can lead to physical dependence and other harmful effects. Although alcohol does help people fall asleep, it also reduces REM and NREM sleep, depriving sleep of much of its restorative power. In addition, nighttime use of alcohol can worsen episodes of early morning awakening as the alcohol is cleared from your body.

Caffeine can also cause sleep problems. Some people are extremely sensitive to even small amounts of caffeine, perhaps because their bodies metabolize it slowly. For these individuals, weak coffee or tea, or even chocolate, can pose a problem if consumed late in the afternoon. Most people learn by experience when to stop their caffeine intake for the day. However, if you are still having trouble sleeping, you might consider eliminating all caffeine-containing products and beverages from your diet.

Exercise

Exercising earlier in the day can improve the quality of your sleep, especially deep, slow-wave, NREM sleep. A 1997 study published in the *Journal of the American Medical Association* showed that elderly people who practiced low-impact aerobic exercise or walked four times a week decreased the time it took them to fall asleep and increased the duration of their sleep.[5]

However, exercising in the evening can be a bad idea if you suffer from insomnia. Exercise temporarily increases your alertness, making it difficult to fall asleep right away.

Sleeping Environment

Your bedroom is another important factor in how well and how long you sleep. Naturally, most of us sleep best in a comfortable, quiet, dark room. Too much light or noise can make it difficult to sleep. Darkness, in fact, actually triggers the release of *melatonin* in the body. Although the exact function of melatonin is still poorly understood, we do know that it aids the body's hormone secretion rhythm.

Exercise temporarily increases your alertness, making it difficult to fall asleep right away.

This rhythm of hormone secretions serves as the body's internal clock, regulating various body functions, including wakefulness and sleepiness (our *circadian rhythm*). Melatonin, then, helps control our periods of wakefulness and sleepiness. Because melatonin release is suppressed by light and stimulated by darkness, keeping the room dark can help us sleep.

When we disturb our circadian rhythm by turning night into day, as occurs with jet lag or changing work shifts, we disrupt the normal rhythmic release and suppression of melatonin, which in turn disrupts our normal sleep cycle.

Another, less obvious factor leading to some people's insomnia is that they use their bed for a wide range of daytime activities. When a bed becomes a place to do homework, watch television, or play games, it can be more difficult to make the mental switch into "sleep mode" at the end of the day.

Worrying About Not Sleeping

Worrying about not sleeping can be a vicious cycle, as it can induce the very thing you're worried about: no sleep. Excessive worrying as a symptom of anxiety was discussed in chapter 2. This annoying cycle of worry, no sleep, anxiety, worry, no sleep, and so on can be broken by relieving the anxiety that precipitates the worrying that causes the sleeplessness.

Conventional Treatment for Insomnia

A comprehensive conventional approach to treating insomnia begins by examining lifestyle factors.[6] Your physician or health-care provider might instruct you to keep a diary for several weeks to learn which factors of diet, exercise, or environment might be contributing to your insomnia. Such diaries usually keep track of when you go to sleep and wake up, when and what you eat, how much alcohol you drink and when, how much you exercise and when, which medications and herbs you take, the sleeping patterns of your bed partner (if you have one), and whether you sleep during the day.

"Do the simple stuff first" is the motto of today's conventional treatment for sleep disorders. Based on the findings of research on sleep and sleep disorders, you might be advised to change many of your sleep habits. You might be instructed to go to sleep only when sleepy rather than lying awake in your bed for hours. You might also be advised to use your bed only for sex and sleep. Such changes are meant to recondition your unconscious responses to your sleeping environment. Daytime sleep should be reduced to no more than one 30-minute nap taken early in the afternoon.

It's also important to keep your bedroom dark and quiet while you sleep. If you read in bed, the lighting should be dim. People who suffer from insomnia should avoid watching television before bedtime because television radiates full-spectrum light.

If such changes in your lifestyle and sleeping environment are not enough to correct your insomnia, your healthcare provider might recommend over-the-counter medication. Modern medical practice recommends the use of the lowest effective dose intermittently (two to four times a week) for short-term use of no more than 3 to 4 weeks. Some sleep aids can cause morning "hangovers" and grogginess, which can lead to memory impairment, falls, accidents, and excessive daytime sleepiness. Because of these side effects, these medications are recommended for temporary use only.

Worrying about not sleeping can begin a vicious cycle, as it can induce the very thing you're worried about: no sleep.

The most common over-the-counter sedatives contain the antihistamines diphenhydramine (Nytol, Sleep-Eze, Sominex) or doxylamine (Unisom, Nighttime), which induce drowsiness.[7] The advantage of these sleep aids is that they're available without prescription. However, they're not for everyone. Individuals with a history of glaucoma, peptic ulcer, or urinary retention should not use them. Antihistamines can also produce unwanted side effects, such as headache, drying of the oral and nasal mucous membranes, nausea, and a feeling of grogginess on awakening.

If you've already made the recommended lifestyle and behavioral changes and the over-the-counter sleep aids don't quite cut it, you might be inclined to ask your physician for a prescription for some sleeping pills. If you do, the prescription you get will most likely be for one of the benzodiazepines, the same class of drugs that includes Valium, Xanax, and other leading antianxiety medications.

For insomnia, the benzodiazepines offer quick, effective relief. Each benzodiazepine affects different stages of sleep, and each differs in the length of time of action— such as short acting or long acting. Your physician will be able assess your sleep patterns and select the right benzodiazepine for you. The medication you're prescribed will depend on whether you have problems falling asleep, whether you wake up in the middle of the night, or whether you awaken too early.

However, as we saw in chapter 4, the benzodiazepines have some drawbacks as well. In the long term, they can potentially become addictive. They can also dramatically alter the normal sleep pattern by reducing REM sleep. This reduction in REM is thought to be a contributing factor to the "morning after" grogginess some people experience when they take benzodiazepine sleeping pills. Even if you don't feel groggy in the morning, your reaction time might be decreased, potentially impairing your driving ability.

A more serious problem is that these medications can induce dependency. Taking them for more than a few days adds a complication called *rebound insomnia.* Simply put, you might have significant trouble sleeping for several days after stopping benzodiazepines. (Again, you should never quit taking a benzodiazepine without a physician's supervision.)

A recent review of 123 controlled medication studies and 33 behavioral interventions for insomnia suggests that both medication and lifestyle/behavioral changes can be effective treatments for insomnia.[8] In the short term, medications were more effective. However, the behavioral changes produced more sustained results. Thus perhaps the best use of medications is for temporary insomnia, whereas changes in behavior and lifestyle offer more relief for chronic insomnia.

Valerian, Kava, and Melatonin for Insomnia

Besides medications, there are several natural treatments for insomnia. As we saw in chapter 9, valerian is sometimes used as a treatment for anxiety. However, it's more commonly recommended as an aid for occasional insomnia. Kava is probably better for anxiety but is sometimes recommended at higher doses to treat insomnia as well. Another natural treatment for insomnia is the hormone melatonin, which (as briefly mentioned) plays an important role in our sleep cycle.

Valerian: An Effective Treatment for Insomnia

Historically, the herb valerian was commonly used for the treatment of insomnia. Although we have some studies that appear to indicate that it is effective, more research is needed to tell us how to use valerian appropriately.

Valerian (*Valeriana officinalis*) is a tall, perennial plant that grows widely in North America, Europe, and Asia. Its root has long been used for medicinal purposes. The Greek physician Galen recommended valerian for insomnia in the second century A.D., and after falling out of common use for some time, it became popular again from the sixteenth century on as a sedative, with wide usage in Europe and the United States. Until 1950, the U.S. National Formulary listed valerian as a sleep aid and antianxiety treatment. However, it fell out of favor once more, as U.S. medical doctors abandoned herbs as a form of treatment.

What Is Valerian Used for Today?

Although valerian lost its place in American medicine after World War II, it continued to be used in Europe. Scientific studies of valerian began in the 1980s, leading to its approval by Germany's Commission E in 1985. Germany's Commission E monograph lists valerian as useful for "restlessness and nervous disturbance of sleep." Today, valerian is available over the counter and is widely used as a remedy for insomnia in Germany, Belgium, France, Switzerland, and Italy. Valerian is considered generally somewhat more effective than the herbs passionflower and hops (see the following discussion) but less effective than pharmaceutical sleeping pills such as the benzodiazepines.

Valerian is once again becoming popular in the United States. Its reputation is as a gentle sleep aid without side effects. As one customer commented, "Valerian is one of the most gentle and harmless herbal sleeping remedies I've found. It seems to enhance my body's natural process of slipping into sleep and makes the stresses of my day recede. I awaken relaxed and refreshed with no morning hangover."

Of course, testimonials such as this one don't prove anything. What we need is evidence, and fortunately there are a few scientific studies we can turn to. However, much remains to be discovered, and valerian's scientific record cannot be regarded as definitive.

What Is the Scientific Evidence for Valerian?

A recent 28-day study of 121 people with a history of sleep disturbances compared the effect of 600 mg of a valerian tincture taken 2 hours before bedtime against placebo. The study concluded that valerian is useful for the long-term treatment of insomnia.[9] Subjects were evaluated by a physician and by self-report at the beginning of the study and at days 14 and 28. At 14 days, no significant differences were found between the two groups' outcomes, but by the end of the fourth week, the group taking valerian showed comparative improvements in quality of sleep, mood, and overall evaluation of results. However, it should be pointed out that the results, although mathematically significant, were not dramatic. Valerian is a very mild treatment.

This study is interesting in that valerian took weeks to achieve its effect. Most people think of valerian as an immediately acting sleeping pill, but this study suggests that it is best used for an extended period of time to improve sleep. However, the picture is a bit confusing, as other studies have found immediate effects. (Interestingly, this is the same situation that exists with kava. The more recent and better designed studies found a slower onset of action than the older ones.)

For example, a double-blind study of 80 elderly individuals with sleep disturbances were given a standardized valerian preparation or placebo for 14 days.[10] The results showed significant improvements compared to placebo on various measures of sleep quality, including time to fall asleep. Similar results have been seen in other studies.[11–13] However, another small study found little to no benefit.[14]

Finally, one very small double-blind study of 20 participants found that 160 mg of valerian root combined with 80 mg of lemon balm (*Melissa officinalis*) was as effective in inducing sleep as 0.125 mg of the benzodiazepine *triazolam* (Halcion).[15] Both drug and herbal combinations were superior to placebo. The herbal treatment enhanced deep, slow-wave sleep without diminishing daytime performance.

Finally, in an enormous open study (one in which the participants knew that they were receiving the treatment), 11,168 individuals with sleep problems reported roughly a 75% improvement in sleep quality after taking a standardized extract for as little as 2 days.[16] Unfortunately, because this was not a controlled or blinded study, it is impossible to eliminate the effects of placebo, and the results can't be taken as meaningful. The lack of side effects seen in this study, however, provides strong evidence that valerian is safe (see discussion following).

Putting all these studies together, it appears that valerian is an effective sleep aid, although conflicting results regarding how fast valerian acts show the need for further research.

What Is in Valerian?

Valerian contains many chemical constituents, including valepotriates, valerenic acid, valeric acid, and isovaleric acid. At one time, it was thought that the important chemical components of valerian were the valepotriates. Now we're not sure exactly which ingredients in valerian are most important. Currently, valerenic acid is being studied, but its role is still unclear.

How Does Valerian Work?

We have only an incomplete understanding of how valerian works. Scientists suggest that valerian affects the brain's levels of gamma-amino-butyric acid (GABA), a naturally occurring amino acid that appears to be related to the experience of anxiety. As you might recall from chapter 4, conventional medications, such as valium, are thought to work by affecting GABA. Studies suggest that valerian either stimulates GABA receptors.[17,18] or increases GABA concentrations.[19] However, these hypotheses have been disputed.[20] Further research is needed to tell us conclusively how valerian works.

Dosage

Valerian is typically taken in tincture, capsule, or tea form, 30 to 60 minutes before bedtime. To be an effective sedative, the tincture form should be taken in dosages of ½ to 2 teaspoons, depending on the concentration.[21] The tea is made by pouring a cup of boiling water over 1 to 3 g of dried root and then left to steep for 10 to 15 minutes. Tablets and capsules are usually taken at a dose of 150 to 300 mg. Standardized extracts should be taken according to label instructions. As with any herb, a good guideline is to start with the smallest dosage first and increase only if needed.

Valerian is seldom effective in individuals who have become habituated to prescription medications for insomnia or anxiety. There is some indication that valerian might be most effective when taken over an extended period of time. Rather than depending on valerian as a crutch, such long-term treatment should be combined with a comprehensive sleep-management program.

Safety Issues

Approved for use as a food, valerian is listed on the U.S. Food and Drug Administration's GRAS (generally regarded as safe) list. Although valerian does not appear to impair driving ability, it can diminish vigilance for a few hours after it's taken. Thus driving a car or operating hazardous machinery within a few hours of taking valerian is not recommended.[22,23]

Aside from its strong odor—some find that valerian root smells unpleasantly like dirty socks—valerian is well tolerated, with only occasional mild gastrointestinal distress. With constant use, side effects can include headaches, excitability, digestive upsets, or sleep and heart disturbances.[24] It is also possible for some people to develop a paradoxical effect from taking valerian, in which valerian actually gives them a mild stimulant effect rather than the expected sedating effect.

No drug interactions have been reported, but the possibility still exists that valerian might enhance other central nervous system depressants, such as sedatives, sleeping pills, and alcohol. As a pharmacist, I recommend erring on the side

> **Valerian is seldom effective in individuals who have become habituated to prescription medications for insomnia or anxiety.**

of safety and not combining valerian with any of these types of medications.

Warning: If you are on any prescription benzodiazepines, do not stop taking them without your physician's advice, as there can be severe consequences.

Safety in young children, pregnant or nursing women, and those with severe liver or kidney disease has not been established.

Kava: Might Help with Insomnia

To recap what we have already learned about kava, it improves sleep by relaxing the body, reducing mental worry and anxiety, and reducing pain. Although no scientific evidence exists that kava can help insomnia, anecdotal stories tell us that traditional healers have prescribed it for insomnia for centuries. Kava-based products are prescribed as medicines for relaxation in France, Germany, Switzerland, and other European countries.

What Is the Scientific Evidence for Kava?

Although we don't have a good definitive study on the effectiveness of kava as a treatment for insomnia, we can look into some studies of kava as an indication that it might be helpful in sleep. A small double-blind placebo-controlled study suggests that synthetic kavain (a kavalactone found in kava) enhances brain activity that favors restorative sleep.[25] At weekly intervals, subjects randomly received placebo; 200, 400, or 600 mg of kavain; or 30 mg of the benzodiazepine Clobazam. Pulse, blood pressure, EEG, psychometric tests, and side effects were noted at the outset and then at 1, 2, 4, 6, and 8 hours after receiving the medication.

EEG activity showed that kavain increased the alpha 1, theta, and delta brain waves that are associated with sleep while decreasing beta waves, which are a sign of wakefulness. Furthermore, these effects increased with higher dosages. At 600 mg, kavain produced sedation comparable to 30 mg of Clobazam.

Unfortunately, this rather theoretical study looked at brain waves rather than true effects on sleep. Also, it used isolated kavain rather than the whole-kava extract as you might purchase it. Much better research needs to be performed before we can say that scientific evidence exists for using kava in sleep disorders.

How Does Kava Work?

The kavalactone components of kava probably account for its reported effects on sleep. Kavalactones pass through the blood-brain barrier and can alter the action of other neurotransmitters (see chapter 5). A sedative and analgesic, kava helps induce sleep in low doses and in high doses, may cause stupor.

Dosage

At bedtime, the recommended dose is 75 to 100 mg of kavalactones; for a stronger sleep-inducing effect, take 150 to 210 mg on an empty stomach.

Safety Issues

The safety of kava is discussed in detail in chapter 7.

Melatonin: A Natural Hormone That Induces Sleep

The body uses the hormone melatonin as part of its normal control of the sleep-wake cycle. The pineal gland—a tiny gland at the base of the brain—makes serotonin and then turns it into melatonin when light decreases. Strong light (such as sunlight) turns off melatonin production. Completely darkened rooms increase melatonin levels more than partially darkened rooms, and weak light doesn't completely shut down melatonin production as does strong light.[26]

Taking melatonin as a supplement seems to stimulate sleep when the natural cycle is disturbed. It's most dramatically effective for jet lag and for those who work night shifts and want to change their hours of sleep on the weekends.

What Is the Scientific Evidence for Melatonin?

One double-blind study enrolled 320 people who were given 5 mg of standard melatonin, 5 mg of slow-release melatonin, 0.5 mg of standard melatonin, or placebo for 4 nights following plane travel.[27] The results showed improvements only with 5 mg of standard melatonin. Benefits were noted in time to fall asleep, quality of sleep, and daytime drowsiness and fatigue.

Positive results were seen in several other studies.[28,29,30] At least one study failed to find a significant sleep-inducing effect for melatonin,[31] but on balance the evidence is strongly positive that melatonin can help sleep.

The body uses the hormone melatonin as part of its normal control of the sleep-wake cycle.

According to one review of the literature, treatment is most effective for those with significant jet lag, such as those who have crossed more than eight time zones.[32] However, melatonin also seems to be help induce sleep for other people, including those with no sleep problems to begin with.

Dosage

Melatonin is typically taken about ½ hour prior to bedtime for the first 4 days after traveling.

The optimum dose of melatonin is not known. It has been suggested that 0.5 mg is the minimum effective dose. However, as noted previously, one study found no effect at 0.5 mg and a positive effect at 5 mg.[33] To further complicate matters, this study also found that only quick-release melatonin was effective. In other studies, time-release forms have been more effective than quick-release forms for helping people sleep through the night. Again, more research is needed to resolve some of these differences in outcomes.

Safety Issues

Melatonin is probably safe for occasional use (as in plane travel), but some real concerns exist about using it on a regular basis. It should be noted that melatonin is not really a food supplement. It is a hormone, just like estrogen, thyroid, or cortisone. It is not a part of your daily diet (unless you are in the habit of eating pineal glands!). Because the body's own production of melatonin is probably the equivalent of only 0.1 mg daily, when you take melatonin for sleep, you are tremendously exceeding the body's own production. The consequences of doing so on a regular basis are completely unknown.[34]

On the basis of theoretical ideas about how melatonin works, some authorities specifically recommend against using it for depression, schizophrenia, autoimmune diseases and other serious illnesses, and in pregnant or nursing women. Do not drive or operate machinery for several hours after taking melatonin.

Other Treatments for Insomnia

In addition to valerian, kava, and melatonin, the herbs passionflower and hops are often used as sleep aids. Other potentially useful herbs for the treatment of insomnia include oat straw, chamomile, lemon balm, catnip, and St. John's wort. However, little to no scientific evidence exists to support their use as sleep aids. Other approaches, such as meditation and biofeedback, might also be useful.

Passionflower

The passionflower vine is a native of the western hemisphere, used by native North Americans mainly as a mild sedative. It quickly caught on as a folk remedy in Europe and thereafter was adopted by professional herbalists as a sedative and digestive aid. Passionflower was recognized officially as a sedative by the U.S. National Formulary from 1916 to 1936. However, in 1978, the U.S. Food and Drug Administration banned it as a sleeping aid for lack of proven effectiveness.

In 1985, Germany's Commission E officially approved passionflower as a treatment for "nervous unrest." The herb is considered to be a mildly effective treatment for anxiety and insomnia—less potent than kava and valerian but useful nonetheless. Like lemon balm, chamomile, and valerian, it is also used for "nervous stomach."

Melatonin is probably safe for occasional use (as in plane travel), but some real concerns exist about using it on a regular basis.

Animal studies suggest that passionflower extracts can prolong sleep and reduce activity levels during wakefulness. However, no double-blind placebo-controlled studies of passionflower in humans have been conducted, except in combination with other herbs.[35]

Several constituents of passionflower have been credited with causing its sedative effect. However, each has been proven ineffective when used alone. At the current state of knowledge, the best we can say is that we don't yet know how (or even if) the herb works.

The proper dose of passionflower is 1 cup 3 times daily of a tea made by steeping 1 teaspoon of dried leaves for 10 to 15 minutes. Passionflower tinctures and powdered extracts should be taken according to the label instructions.

Passionflower is on the U.S. Food and Drug Administration's GRAS list. Although the alkaloids harman and harmaline found in passionflower can increase the effects of MAO inhibitors and also stimulate the uterus,[36] it seems unlikely that the use of normal doses of passionflower presents the same risks.

Safety has not been established for young children, pregnant or nursing mothers, and those with severe liver or kidney disease.

Hops

As we saw in chapter 9, hops (the flowering part of the hops plant) are most famous as the source of beer's bitter flavor, but they also have a long history of use in herbal medicine. In Greece and Rome, hops were used as a remedy for poor digestion and intestinal disturbances. The Chinese used the herb for these purposes and to treat leprosy and tuberculosis.

Studies show that meditative relaxation, biofeedback, and progressive muscle relaxation techniques can also be useful to help promote sleep.

As cultivation of hops for beer spread through Europe, it gradually became obvious that workers in hops fields tended to fall asleep on the job, more so than could be explained by the tedium of the work. This observation led to enthusiasm for using hops as a sedative. However, subsequent investigation suggests that much of the sedative effect seen in hops fields is due to an oil that evaporates quickly during storage.

Nonetheless, dried hops preparations do appear to be somewhat calming. Although the exact reason is not clear, it seems that a sedating substance known as methyl-butenol develops in the dried herb over a period of time. It can also be manufactured in the body from other constituents of hops.

Germany's Commission E authorizes the use of hops for "discomfort due to restlessness or anxiety and sleep disturbances." Scientists have had difficulty demonstrating that hops causes sedation, probably because the effect is so mild.[37] The herb is often combined with other treatments. Like other bitter plants, hops can also improve appetite and digestion.

The standard dose of hops is 0.5 g taken 1 to 3 times daily.

Hops are believed to be nontoxic. However, as with all herbs, some people are allergic to it. Interestingly, some species of dogs, especially greyhounds, appear to be sensitive to hops; in fact, some canine deaths have been reported.[38] The mechanism of this toxicity is not yet known. Hobbyists who brew their own beer are advised to keep pets away from the relatively large quantity of hops used in this process.

Safety in young children, pregnant or nursing women, and those with severe liver or kidney disease has not been established.

Lifestyle Changes

The following is a reminder for you as you consider lifestyle changes that might help with your sleep habits.

- Exercise earlier in the day.
- Lower or eliminate alcohol and caffeine consumption.
- Darken your bedroom or wear an eyeshade.
- Lessen noise by wearing earplugs or use a "white noise" machine, which provides a nondescript background

noise that tends to blend bothersome sounds into the background.

- Use your bed only for sleeping or sex.
- Try changing pillows to fit your body's individual comfort needs; likewise, make sure that your mattress is comfortable.
- Control body temperature to induce sleep. If you're too warm, your movement increases; if you're too cold, you awaken more.

Mind-Body Behavioral Approaches

Studies show that meditative relaxation, biofeedback, and progressive muscle relaxation techniques can also be useful to help promote sleep. A 12-member panel representing family medicine, psychiatry, public health, nursing, and epidemiology met at the National Institutes of Health with 23 experts in behavioral and sleep medicine to discuss new approaches to insomnia and pain. Their findings indicate that relaxation techniques and biofeedback are effective in treating insomnia. Cognitive forms of relaxation, such as meditation, are slightly better than somatic forms, such as progressive muscle relaxation. Although all these techniques are useful, the panel concluded that the success of any of these techniques for improving sleep requires that you take responsibility for learning and practicing them.[39] However, the great advantage of these techniques is that they can help improve other areas of your life as well.

A Relaxing Combination

Using kava or valerian in combination with a mind-body relaxation technique, plus ensuring that the bedroom environment is dark and quiet, can help eliminate your insomnia. Another relaxing option is to sip a tea of passionflower and hops and listen to soft music in a candlelit room for 1 to 2 hours before bedtime to condition your body to relax and expect a gentle, restoring sleep.

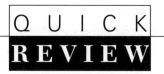

- Insomnia compromises our health and well-being in many ways.
- Lack of sleep can make us feel anxious or depressed while depleting the brain's stores of energy.
- Our cognitive functioning and performance suffer when we are chronically short of sleep. Insomnia also impairs our immune system.
- Prescription and over-the-counter medications are useful tools with which to treat insomnia. They work fast and are generally effective. However, the side effects of these treatments include dependence and morning grogginess.
- Although some research exists on the effectiveness of valerian for treating insomnia, more investigation is needed. For sleep, valerian tincture should be taken in dosages of ½ to 2 teaspoonfuls, 30 to 60 minutes before bedtime. Tablets and capsules are usually taken at a dosage of 150 to 300 mg; standardized extracts should be taken according to label instructions.
- Some studies indicate that valerian is effective immediately, whereas others suggest that 4 weeks of steady usage are necessary for full effects.
- No direct evidence has been found that kava can improve insomnia, but it's widely used for this purpose. At bedtime, the recommended dose is 75 to 210 mg of kavalactones.

- Research has found that the use of melatonin as a supplement seems to stimulate sleep, but its safety when used on a daily basis is questionable.

- Other herbal remedies widely used for insomnia include passionflower and hops.

- Lifestyle factors and mind-body behavior approaches can be practiced in combination with herbs or medications.

Putting It All Together

For your easy reference, this chapter contains a brief summary of key information contained in this book. Please refer to earlier chapters for more comprehensive information, including a detailed discussion of safety issues.

If you are suffering from mild to moderate anxiety, kava may offer an effective alternative to prescription medications. Consult with your physician first to make sure you don't have a serious medical problem that needs more specific treatment.

To treat anxiety, the usual daily dose of kava should supply 20 to 70 mg of kavalactones 3 times daily. The total dose of kavalactones should not exceed 300 mg daily, and the course of treatment should not exceed 3 months. The full antianxiety effects may take from 4 to 8 weeks to develop in some cases; however, you may experience more immediate relief.

Kava appears to be safe when taken in the usual dosages. Some cases of dermopathy (skin rash) have been reported in people taking very high dosages over a long period of time, but there doesn't seem to be any cause for alarm—the rash isn't dangerous, and it hasn't been reported at the dosages used in Europe or North America. Do not combine kava with alcohol or other drugs that depress the central nervous system, because the overall effect may be extreme and possibly dangerous sedation. And, as with most other herbs and drugs, kava's safety in children and pregnant or nursing mothers has not been established. We also don't know if kava continues to be safe when taken in the long term. This is the reason why kava is only recommended for use over a 3-month period.

Other Natural Treatments for Anxiety

If kava does not help you with your symptoms of anxiety, there are other natural treatments that might help. Valerian is another safe herbal alternative that is also suggested as a treatment for anxiety taken at a dosage of 2 to 3 g twice daily. However, there is little scientific evidence on its effectiveness for anxiety. It is more commonly used for insomnia (see following).

Other herbs sometimes recommended for anxiety include lemon balm, hops, skullcap, and lady's slipper. However, there is next to no evidence that they are effective. Whereas lemon balm and hops are believed to be safe when used in reasonable doses, the safety of skullcap and lady's slipper has not been established.

Other supplements, such as GABA, selenium, flaxseed oil, and multivitamins, have been suggested as aids for treating anxiety, but there is no scientific evidence at this time on the effectiveness of these remedies.

Lifestyle changes can help improve the external factors that can fuel anxiety and add to our overall health. Psychotherapy is an important therapeutic tool for those whose anxiety has a basis in emotional conflicts. These tools require commitment and time but can give lasting, wide-ranging benefits. They can also be an important addition to any medications or herbs you are taking.

Other Natural Treatments for Insomnia

Insomnia is closely connected to anxiety, and can sap your energy and weaken your immune system. Evidence suggests that the herb **valerian** can improve sleep, especially when taken for many weeks in a row. For sleep, valerian tincture should be taken in dosages of ½ to 2 teaspoonfuls, 30 to 60 minutes before bedtime. Tablets and capsules are usually taken at a dosage of 150 to 300 mg; standardized extracts should be taken according to label instructions.

No direct evidence has been found that kava can improve insomnia, but it's widely used for this purpose. At bedtime, the recommended dose is 75 to 210 mg of kavalactones.

Research has found that the use of **melatonin** as a supplement seems to stimulate sleep, but its safety when used on a daily basis is questionable.

Other herbal remedies widely used for insomnia include **passionflower** and **hops.** Lifestyle factors and mind-body behavior approaches can be practiced in combination with herbs or medications.

Finally, if you suffer from severe anxiety or insomnia, don't be close-minded to the possibility of taking prescription medications. They can be quite safe and effective when used properly.

Notes

Chapter Five

1. Warnecke G, et al. Wirksamkeit von kawa-kawa-extract beim klimakterischen syndrom. *Z Phytother* 11: 81–86, 1990. [Cited in Schulz V, et al. Rational phytotherapy. New York: Springer-Verlag, 1998: 71.]

2. Warnecke G. Neurovegetative dystonia in the female climacteric. Studies on the clinical efficacy and tolerance of kava extract WS -1490. *Fortschr Med* 109: 119–122, 1991.

3. Kinzler E, et al. Clinical efficacy of a kava extract in patients with anxiety syndrome of non-psychotic origin. Double-blind placebo controlled study over 4 weeks. *Arzneim-Forsch/Drug Res* 41: 584–88, 1991.

4. Volz HP and Kieser M. Kava-kava extract WS 1490 versus placebo in anxiety disorders—a randomized placebo-controlled 25-week outpatient trial. *Pharmacopsychiat* 30: 1–5, 1997.

5. Volz HP and Kieser M. 1997.

6. Warnecke G. 1991.

7. Warnecke G, et al. 1990.

8. Kinzler E, et al. 1991.

9. Lehmann E, et al. Efficacy of a special kava extract *(Piper methysticum)* in patients with states of anxiety, tension and excitedness of non-mental origin: a double-blind placebo-controlled study of four weeks duration. *Phytomedicine* 3: 113–119, 1996.

10. Singh N, et al. A double-blind, placebo controlled study on the effects of kava (Kavatrol) on daily stress and anxiety in

adults. Unpublished study from Virginia Commonwealth University, Richmond, VA.

11. Schulz V, et al. Rational phytotherapy. New York: Springer-Verlag, 1998: 71.

12. Schulz, V. 1998.

13. Davies L, et al. Effects of kava on benzodiazepine and GABA receptor binding. *Europ J Pharmacol* 183: 558, 1990.

14. Jussofie A, et al. Kavapyrone enriched extract from *Piper methysticum* as modulator of the GABA binding site in different regions of rat brain. *Psychopharmacology* 116: 469–474, 1994.

15. Gleitz J, et al. (+)-Kavain inhibits veratridine-activated voltage-dependent Na+ channels in synaptosomes prepared from rat cerebral cortex. *Neuropharmacology* 34(9): 1133–1138, 1995.

16. Gleitz J, et al. Kavain inhibits non-stereospecifically veratridine-activated Na+ channels. *Planta Med* 62: 580–581, 1996.

Chapter Six

1. Schulz V, et al. Rational phytotherapy. New York: Springer-Verlag, 1998: 71.

Chapter Seven

1. Schulz V, et al. Rational phytotherapy. New York: Springer-Verlag, 1998: 71.

2. Schulz, V et al. 1998.

3. Schulz V et al. 1998.

4. Norton SL and Ruse P. Kava dermopathy. *Journal of the American Academy of Dermatology,* 31(1): 89–96, 1994.

5. Schelosky L, Raffauf C, and Jendroska K, et al. W. Poewe of the neurology department at Rudolph Virehote University in Berlin.(letter). *J Neurol Neurosurg Psychiatry* 45: 639–640, 1995.

6. Meyer HJ. Pharmakologie der Wirksamen Prinzipien des Kawa-Rhizoms (*Piper methysticum* Forst). *Arch Int Pharmacodyn Ther* 138: 505–535. Cited in Bone K. (1995). Kava-Kava—A safe herbal treatment for anxiety. *Townshend Letter for Doctors.* June 1995: 85.

7. Jamieson DD and Duffield PH. Positive interaction of ethanol and kava resin in mice. *Clinical and Experimental Pharmacology and Physiology* 17: 509–514, 1990.

8. Swensen J. Man convicted of driving under influence of kava. *Desert News* (Salt Lake City, UT), August 5, 1996.

9. Mathews J, et al. Effects of the heavy usage of kava on physical health: summary of a pilot survey in an Aboriginal community. *The Medical Journal of Australia* 148: 548–555, 1988.

10. Duffield AM and Jamieson DD. Development of tolerance to kava in mice. *Clinical and Experimental Pharmacology and Physiology* 18: 571–578, 1991.

11. Almeida JC and Grimsley EW. Coma from the health food store: Interaction between kava and alprazolam. *Ann Intern Med* 125(11): 940, 1996.

12. Jamieson DD and Duffield PH. 1990.

Chapter Eight

1. Woelk H, et al. The treatment of patients with anxiety. A double blind study: kava extract WS 1490 vs. benzodiazepine. *Zitschrift fur Allgemenie Medizine* 69: 271–77, 1993.

2. Lindenberg V and Pitule-Schodel H. Dl-kavain im vergleich zu oxazepam bei angstzustanden. *Fortschr Med* 108: Jg., 1990.

3. Schulz V, et al. Rational phytotherapy. New York: Springer-Verlag, 1998: 70.

4. Munte TF, et al. Effects of oxazepam and an extract of kava roots *(Piper methysticum)* on event-related potentials in a word recognition task. *Neuropsychobiology* 27(1): 46–53, 1993.

5. Heinze HJ, et al. Pharmacopsychological effects of oxazepam and kava-extract in a visual search paradigm assessed with event-related potentials. *Pharmacopsychiatry* 27(6): 224–230, 1994.

Chapter Nine

1. Holzl J, et al. Receptor binding studies with *Valeriana officinalis* on the benzodiazepine receptor. *Planta Med* 55: 642, 1989.

2. Mennini T, et al. in vitro study on the interaction of extracts and pure compounds from *Veleriana officinalis* roots with

GABA, benzodiazepine and barbiturate receptors in rat brain. *Fitoterapia* 54: 291–300, 1993.

3. Schulz V, et al. Rational phytotherapy. New York: Springer-Verlag, 1998: 75–76.

4. Cavadas C, et al. In vitro study on the interaction of *Valeriana officinalis* L. extracts and their amino acids on GABAA receptor in rat brain. *Arzneimittelforschung* 45(7): 753–755, 1995.

5. Kohnen R, et al. the effects of valerian, propranolol, and their combination in activation, performance and mood of healthy volunteers under social stress conditions. *Pharmacopsychiatry* 21(6): 447–448, 1988.

6. ESCOP monographs. Fascicule 4: *Valerianae radix* (valerian). Exeter, UK: European Scientific Cooperative on Phytotherapy, 1997: 2.

Chapter Ten

1. Coren S. Sleep thieves. New York, NY: Simon & Schuster, Inc., 1996.

2. Kupder DJ and Reynolds CF. Current concepts: management of insomnia. *New England Journal of Medicine,* 336(5)341–346, 1997.

3. Coren S. 1996.

4. Kupder DJ and Reynolds CF. 1997.

5. King AC, et al. Moderate-intensity exercise and self-rated quality of sleep in older adults. *Journal of the American Medical Assoc* 277: 32–37, 1997.

6. King. 1997.

7. Murray M. Stress, anxiety, and insomnia. Rocklin, CA: Prima Publishing, 1995.

8. NIH Technology Assessment Panel on Integration of Behavioral and Relaxation Approaches into the Treatment of Chronic Pain and Insomnia. *Journal of the American Medical Assoc* 276: 24–31, 1996.

9. Schulz V, et al. Rational phytotherapy. New York: Springer-Verlag, 1998: 78–80.

10. Kamm-Kohl AV, et al. Modern valerian therapy of nervous disorders in elderly patients. *Medwelt* 35: 1450–1454, 1984.

11. Leathwood PD, et al. Aqueous extract of valerian root *(Valeriana officinalis L.)* improves sleep quality in man. *Pharmacol Biochem Behav* 17(1): 65–71, 1982.

12. Leathwood PD, et al. Aqueous extract of valerian reduces latency to fall asleep in man. *Planta Med* 51: 144–148, 1985.

13. Lindahl O, et al. Double blind study of a valerian preparation. *Pharmacol Biochem Behav* 32(4): 1065–1066, 1989.

14. Schulz H, et al. The effect of valerian extract on sleep polygraphy in poor sleepers: a pilot study. *Pharmacopsychiatry* 27: 147–51, 1994.

15. Dressing H, et al. Insomnia: are valeriana and melissa combinations of equal value to benzodiazepine? *Therpiewoche* 42: 726–736. 1992.

16. Schmidt-Voigt J. Treatment of nervous sleep disturbances and inner restlessness with a purely herbal sedative: results of a study in general practice. *Therapiewoche* 36: 663–667, 1986.

17. Holzl J, et al. Receptor binding studies with *Valeriana officinalis* on the benzodiazepine receptor. *Planta Med* 55: 642, 1989.

18. Mennini T, et al. in vitro study on the interaction of extracts and pure compounds from *Veleriana officinalis* roots with GABA, benzodiazepine and barbiturate receptors in rat brain. *Fitoterapia* 54: 291–300, 1993.

19. Schulz V. 1998: 75–76.

20. Santos MS, et al. III The amount of GABA present in aqueous extracts of valerian is sufficient to account for [^{3}H] GABA release in synaptosomes. *Planta Med* 60: 475–476, 1994.

21. Hoffman David. The elements of herbalism. Longmead, Dorset, UK: Element Books, 1990: 24–28.

22. Albrecht M, et al. Psychopharmaceuticals and safety in traffic. *Z Allg Med* 71: 1215–1221, 1995.

23. Gerhard U, et al. Vigilance-decreasing effects of 2 plant-derived sedatives. *Schweiz Rundsch Med Prax* 85: 473–481, 1996.

24. Hobbs C. Valerian: a literature review. *Herbalgram* 21: 19–34, 1989.

25. Saletu B. et al. G brain mapping, psychometric and psychophysiological studies on central effects of kavain. *Human Psychopharmacology* 4: 169–190, 1989.

26. Lamberg L. Melatonin potentially useful but safety, efficacy remain uncertain. *JAMA* 276(13): 1011–1014, 1996.

27. Suhner A, et al. Optimal melatonin dosage form for the alleviation of jet lag. *Chronobiol Int* 14: 41, 1997.

28. Garfinkel D, et al. Improvement of sleep quality in elderly people by controlled-release melatonin. *Lancet* 346: 541–544, 1995.

29. Petrie K, et al. A double-blind trial of melatonin as a treatment for jet lag in international cabin crew. *Bio Psych* 33(7): 526–530, 1993.

30. Chase JE, et al. Melatonin: therapeutic use in sleep disorders. *Ann Pharmacother* 346(10): 1218–1226, 1997.

31. Spitzer RL, et al. Failure of melatonin to affect jet lag in a randomized double blind trial. *Soc Light Treatment Biol Rhythms Abstr* 9: 1, 1997.

32. Arendt J, et al. Efficacy of melatonin in jet lag, shift work and blindness. *J Bio Rhythms* 12 (6): 604–617, 1997.

33. Suhner A, et al. Optimal melatonin dosage form for the alleviation of jet lag. *Chronobiol Int* 14: 41, 1997.

34. Waterhouse J, et al. Jet Lag. *Lancet* 350: 1611–1616, 1997.

35. Schulz V. 1998: 84.

36. Newall C, Anderson L, and Phillipson J. Herbal medicines: a guide for health-care professionals. London: The pharmaceutical press, 1996: 206.

37. Schulz V. 1998: 83.

38. Duncan KL, et al. Malignant hyperthermia-like reaction secondary to ingestion of hops in five dogs. *J Am Vet Med Assoc* 210: 51–54, 1997.

39. NIH Technology Assessment Panel on Integration of Behavioral and Relaxation Approaches into the Treatment of Chronic Pain and Insomnia. *Journal of the American Medical Assoc* 276: 24–31, 1996.

Index

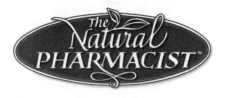

About the Author

Constance Grauds, R.Ph., is president of the Association of Natural Medicine Pharmacists, whose mission statement is to provide pharmacist education and certification on natural medicines. She is assistant clinical pharmacy professor at the University of California at Berkeley and writes for *Pharmacy Times* and *Review of Natural Products.*

About the Series Editors

Steven Bratman, M.D., medical director of Prima Health, has many years of experience in the alternative medicine field. A graduate of the University of California at Davis, Medical School, he has also trained in herbology, nutrition, Chinese medicine, and other alternative therapies, and has worked closely with a wide variety of alternative practitioners. He is the author of *The Natural Pharmacist: Your Complete Guide to Herbs* (Prima), *The Natural Pharmacist: Your Complete Guide to Illnesses and Their Natural Remedies* (Prima), *The Natural Pharmacist Guide to St. John's Wort and Depression* (Prima), *The Alternative Medicine Ratings Guide* (Prima), and *The Alternative Medicine Sourcebook* (Lowell House).

David J. Kroll, Ph.D., is a professor of pharmacology and toxicology at the University of Colorado School of Pharmacy and a consultant for pharmacists, physicians, and alternative practitioners on the indications and cautions for herbal medicine use. A graduate of both the University of Florida and the Philadelphia College of Pharmacy and Science, Dr. Kroll has lectured widely and has published articles in a number of medical journals, abstracts, and newsletters.